High-Risk Newborn Home Care Manual

High-Risk Newborn Home Care Manual

Mary Ann Chestnut, RN

President, Citadel MCH, Inc.
Narberth, Pennsylvania

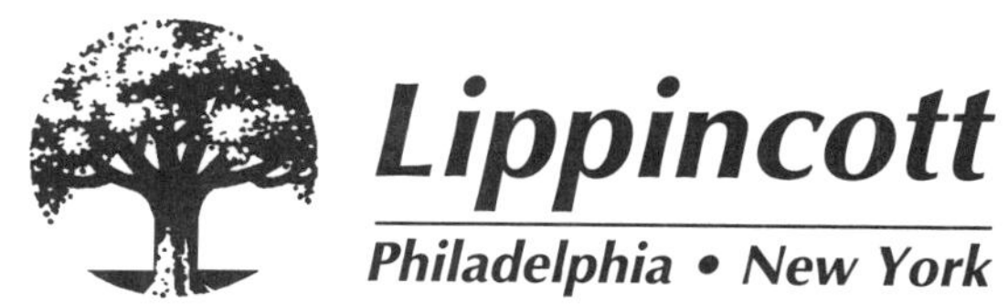

Lippincott
Philadelphia • New York

Acquisitions Editor: Jennifer E. Brogan
Coordinating Editorial Assistant: Susan V. Barta
Production Editor: Virginia Barishek
Production Manager: Helen Ewan
Production Service: Berliner Inc.
Printer/Binder: Victor Graphics
Cover Designer: Joan Wendt
Cover Printer: Lehigh Press

9   8   7   6   5   4   3   2   1

Library of Congress Cataloging-in-Publication Data
   Chestnut, Mary Ann
     High-risk newborn home care manual / Mary Ann Chestnut.
        p.   cm.
     Includes bibliographical references and index.
     ISBN 0-397-55477-X
     1. Infants (Newborn)—Home care—Handbooks, manuals, etc.
  2. Infants (Newborn)—Diseases—Nursing—Handbooks, manuals, etc.
  I. Title.
     [DNLM: 1. Neonatal Nursing—methods.   2. Home Care Services—
  standards.   WY 157 C525h 1997]
  RJ255.C53   1997
  618.92'01—dc21
  DNLM/DLC
  for Library of Congress   97-25844
                                          CIP

Care has been taken to confirm the accuracy of the information presented and to describe generally accepted practices. However, the authors, editors, and publisher are not responsible for errors or omissions or for any consequences from application of the information in this book and make no warranty, express or implied, with respect to the contents of the publication.

The authors, editors and publisher have exerted every effort to ensure that drug selection and dosage set forth in this text are in accordance with current recommendations and practice at the time of publication. However, in view of ongoing research, changes in government regulations, and the constant flow of information relating to drug therapy and drug reactions, the reader is urged to check the package insert for each drug for any change in indications and dosages and for added warnings and precautions. This is particularly important when the recommended agent is a new or infrequently employed drug.

Some drugs and medical devices presented in this publication have Food and Drug Administration (FDA) clearance for limited use in restricted research settings. It is the responsibility of the health care provider to ascertain the FDA status of each drug or device planned for use in their clinical practice.

— To Paul Branca, M.D. —

Until his death in 1989, Dr. Branca was the Director of Neonatology at Thomas Jefferson University Hospital in Philadelphia, where he aggressively supported the art and science of nursing. He challenged this nurse to create a home health service dedicated to maternal–child care.

To this day I thank him for reminding me that "It is easy to follow existing health care standards, the challenge is creating new and better ones."

Preface

Throughout this century American society has continually reaffirmed its concern for the health and well-being of its mothers, infants, and children. Initiatives to reduce infant mortality have included efforts to improve prenatal care, increase coordination between services, and provide more comprehensive services. Infants born with medical problems have special health care needs that mandate efforts to provide and coordinate comprehensive services. These include medical, social support, nutrition, and educational services. The very first White House Conference convened in 1909 by President Theodore Roosevelt emphasized the importance of comprehensive health services for mothers and infants.

Families of infants with special health needs require an evaluation of the need for home health nursing support as an important component of comprehensive services. Home health services for children seek to identify and resolve problems that may increase the risks of morbidity and mortality while also providing interventions specific to an existing medical problem. *The High-Risk Newborn Home Care Manual* is the result of 12 years of research and practical applications. This book can be used by all those responsible—home health providers, discharge planners, nurse educators, managed care providers, nurses working in the field, and physicians—to assure quality, comprehensive care to newborns.

Chapter 1 includes the personnel policies necessary to assure standards for recruitment, experience, and performance of nurses working in the field. Chapter 2 offers standards to assess psychosocial problems which, if present, may increase the risks for morbidity and mortality. These factors include life transitions; emotional status; substance abuse and risk-taking behaviors; parenting issues; educational and cultural issues; economic and resource needs; and maternal and infant medical, nutritional, and environmental factors. This chapter also provides a complete review of standards for the physical assessment of the newborn. Included are those findings considered to be within normal limits, along with deviations and resultant actions to follow. Providers of care will find these helpful tools for reference in the field.

Chapter 3 describes standards that may be included in a comprehensive follow-up program of home visits for the high-risk newborn. The psychosocial and physical standards provided in Chapter 2 are used to identify a level of risk and to establish a goal-oriented plan of care that is accomplished through a series of regularly scheduled home visits throughout the first year of life. These standards were developed based upon recommendations published by several federal task forces and commissions organized to study the prevention of infant morbidity and mortality. These include the Federal Task Force to Study and Make Recommendations on the Content of Prenatal Care, the National Commission to Prevent Infant Mortality, and the National Institutes of Health Committee to Study the Prevention of Low Birthweight.

Chapter 4 contains policies and procedures for the performance of invasive procedures in the home. Procedures for obtaining blood specimens and starting, maintaining, and discontinuing peripheral intravenous therapy are described. Chapter 5 details nursing protocols for specific health problems often encountered in home care. These protocols include apnea monitoring, prematurity, failure to thrive, oxygen administration, seizure disorders, and colostomy care. A common reason for hospital admissions of children (more than 200,000 annually) is treatment of complications of diarrhea. With that statistic in mind, this chapter also includes a home visiting program developed for use in the author's home health agency and in accordance with guidelines from the Johns Hopkins University's Oral Rehydration Program.

Chapter 6 provides educational materials that may be copied and distributed to clients and their families for teaching and reference. Visual and written aids enhance the education process for the client, especially when the nurse reviews the materials with the client.

The Appendix contains additional useful information. It includes home visiting forms that can be utilized as clinical records. These forms have been used in the author's programs that have secured both Medicare certification and accreditation by the Joint Commission on the Accreditation of Healthcare Organizations (JCAHO). These forms have also been designed to help collect standard data necessary to evaluate services and outcomes. There is also a glossary, a list of common abbreviations, and a bibliography. All providers of maternal–child home health services should have at least a small reference library; the bibliography will be helpful in developing such a resource.

Mary Ann Chestnut, RN

Acknowledgments

As a nurse working in the field of maternal–child health since 1982, I have had the privilege of working with many individuals who contributed to my knowledge and inspired me to write and publish this manuscript. I would like to thank and acknowledge those who have so willingly contributed this support.

- *The staff of Booth Maternity Center, Philadelphia, Pennsylvania, who are too numerous to list here.*

- *The staff at Family Help, Inc., including:*
    Ellen Craighead, RN, BSN
    Marilyn Kerr, RN, BSN
    Bonnie Charleston
    Anne Ravdin, RN, BSN
    Ann Galanter, RN, BSN
    Joanne Fischer, MSW
    Laurie Reardon, RN, BSN
    Barbara Tinus, RN, BSN
    Gail Pierson, RN, PNP
    Barbara Krinsky, RN, BSN
    Millie Boettcher, RN, MSN
    Patricia Larsen, RN, MSN, CNM
    Debbie Westcott, RN, BSN
    Judy Woomer, CHHA
    and all the other staff who made Family
    Help a reality

- *The staff at Citadel MCH Services*
    Sonya Newell Wilson, RN
    Kathleen Whalen, RN
    Jacqueline Williams, RN, BSN
    Vicki Newell
    Carol Hallenback, RN, BSN
    Judy Podosky, RNC
    Ann Galanter, RN, BS
    Norma Cintron, RN

Paul Branca, MD
Ronald Bolognese, MD
Judy Bernbaum, MD
Evelyn Bouden, MD
Carl Bailey
Jannie L. Blackwell
Roberta Capewell, RN, MSN, PNP
Julia Clarke, RN, CNM, MSN
Jane Eleey, MSW
Jeffrey Gerdes, MD
Page Talbott Gould, PhD
Howard Grant, MD, JD
Robert Holmes, MD
Susan Hutchinson, RNC, MSN
Mark A. Kalchbrenner, DO
Rich Kaplan, MD
June Kinney, PhD
Rose Kinney, RN, BSN
Judith McCoyd, ACSW, LSW
Carol L. Natter, PT
Lucille Pema, RN, BSN
Albert Pizzica, DO
Barbara Ritchey, ACSW, LSW
Jeffrey Rothirtan, EdD:, PT
Barbara Schraeder, RN, PhD
Robert Stavis, PhD, MD
Patricia Thiebault, RD
Barbara Wesley, MD, MPH
Robert S. Wimmer, MD
Mary Wright, MOT
Susan Yates, CNM, MSN

- *Also a joint acknowledgment must be made to those who served on The Professional Advisory Committees of Family Help, Inc. (1985–1990) and/or The Professional Advisory Committees of Citadel MCH Services, Inc. (1991–1995):*

- *I also want to thank Scott Bucher, RN and Mylo Woodward, RN of the Pennsylvania Department of Health, Maternal–Child Division, and Frank Heron of the U.S. Department of Health and Human Services for their support and assistance throughout the years.*

Contents

■ CHAPTER 5

Specific Protocols for High-Risk Newborn Follow-Up   53

■ CHAPTER 6

Family Education Materials   109

Bibliography   139

Appendices   145

High-Risk Newborn
Home Care Manual

Personnel Policies and Procedures

This chapter covers the personnel policies and procedures relative to nursing performance when making high-risk newborn nursing home visits. Administrative persons will find these helpful for job description purposes. All nurses either supervising or providing direct care should be provided with a copy of this section during orientation in order to understand performance requirements adequately. In addition, these standards should be used as a component of concurrent and retrospective audits for quality of services rendered. These standards will also provide a means to assess comprehensive nursing practice as part of the evaluation process for nurses working within the program.

■ STANDARD NURSING PRACTICE

PURPOSE: These guidelines are designed to apply uniform quality standards in professional nursing practice related to the high-risk newborn visit within the family-centered care program.

RATIONALE: Guidelines are provided for the professional employee for expected standards of practice within the family-centered care program.

RESPONSIBLE TO: The nurse participating in the family-centered care program is responsible to the Director of Nursing.

CONTENT: The duties and responsibilities of the nurse in the family-centered care program are described below.

1. Receives and records the clinical assignment from the supervisor.

2. Verifies the time of the scheduled visit with the client before arrival.

3. Establishes a client relationship using the "helping relationship" (orientation, working, and termination stages) (Box 1-1).

4. Reviews Terms and Conditions of Services, including requirements for third-party reimbursement, with the client before beginning work.

5. Explains all procedures and rationales to the client before performance.

6. Reviews normal newborn behavior (types of crying, sleeping patterns, stimulation, and bonding).

7. Discusses self-care measures necessary to the family of the high-risk newborn, employing the concept of active decision making by the client in relation to self-care needs.

8. Practices a preventive approach to depression using key causative factors and troubleshooting methods. Depression can be brought on by the stress of a high-risk newborn.

9. Evaluates for the need of Home Health Aide services or evaluates the services if they are being utilized.

10. Reviews community resources available to the family (insurance coverage, health clinics, breastfeeding groups, parenting groups, etc.).

11. Provides preventive health teaching concerning early intervention programs, the effects of secondhand smoke on the newborn, diet, infant immunizations, the need for physical examinations, signs and symptoms of illness in the family and baby, and resuscitative and emergency procedures for newborns.

12. Performs assessment of newborn, checking appearance, skin color, heart rate and sounds, temperature, respiratory rate and character, neurologic status, muscle tone, abdomen, neck, extremities, femoral pulse, genitalia, history of voiding and bowel movement, condition of umbilicus, condition of circumcision if new, nutritional history from birth, and current nutrition.

BOX 1-1: THE HELPING RELATIONSHIP

Orientation Phase: The client will know the nurse by name and accurately describe the roles of the participants in the relationship. The client and nurse will establish an agreement regarding:

- Goals of the relationship
- Location, frequency, and length of contact

Working Phase: The nurse and client work together to meet the client's goals. The client actively participates, cooperating in activities to reach those goals. The client can express his or her feelings and concerns to the nurse.

Termination: The client participates in identifying progress toward or accomplishment of goals. The client verbalizes feelings about the termination of the relationship.

---

13. Provides instruction in newborn care with each home visit, covering bathing, cord care, diapering and dressing, diaper rash, circumcision care, fresh air, stuffy nose, sleeping, visiting, immunizations, medications, books available, cool mist, temperature-taking techniques, ipecac, meeting the infant's physical and emotional needs, and problems that require special attention.

14. Reviews patient education materials.

■ HIGH-RISK NEWBORN ASSESSMENT

POLICY: A newborn assessment will be performed on all clients referred to the high-risk newborn program.

PURPOSE: The newborn assessment is conducted to provide nursing assessment for newborns within the first days after hospital discharge.

PROCEDURE: The procedures to be used for conducting the newborn assessment are described below.

1. The hospital will assure that all infants receive access to home visiting nurse services after discharge.

2. The agency or nurse will contact the mother after the referral is received.

3. A visit will be scheduled according to the plan of care.

4. If the nurse is unable to schedule a visit, the nurse will contact the agency about the problem, within the first 24 hours after discharge. The agency will notify the hospital care provider and insurer (if required).

5. If the mother and infant are not at home when the nurse arrives for the visit, the nurse will contact the agency with a report on the status of the visit and will continue to attempt to see the baby based upon additional information the agency, hospital nurse, or insurer is able to provide.

6. The nurse will obtain a signed consent from the mother/guardian for the baby as required.

7. The nurse will perform a physical assessment of the newborn.

8. The nurse will perform a risk assessment and determine whether there are problems requiring additional home care or follow-up by the health care provider.

9. The nurse will complete the Newborn Universal Home Risk Assessment tool for the baby, clearly noting the mother's insurance number and type, date of birth, WIC appointment, baby's pediatric health care provider, the date and time of the follow-up appointment, and all other required information.

10. The nurse will also assess the client's awareness of high-risk newborn programs and services offered by the community, the insurer, the local department of health, or early intervention programs. The nurse should assist in identifying appropriate services for the infant.

11. The nurse will review emergency numbers and safety measures with the mother.

12. The nurse will make referrals to other agencies as needed.

13. The nurse will have the mother sign a time log for her baby.

14. The nurse will notify the agency when the assessment has been completed and will report whether or not the patient will be referred into the home care program.

15. The nurse will return the completed assessments, consent forms, and time logs to the agency.

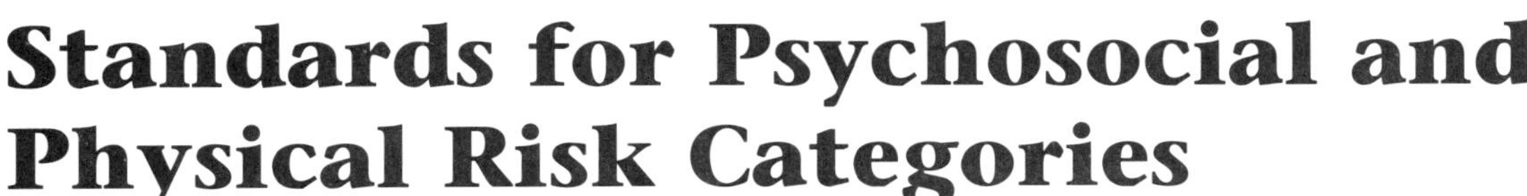

CHAPTER 2

Standards for Psychosocial and Physical Risk Categories

As more complex and alternative care is being provided in the home, resources must exist to help caregivers respond to this growing need. This manual was developed to provide such a tool. "Home visiting has been shown to be an effective means of reducing infant mortality" (National Commission to Prevent Infant Mortality). Identification and evaluation of the high-risk newborn ideally begins in the prenatal period and is an ongoing process. The infant must be assessed at birth and again at various points thereafter given the findings during the first year of life.

To assure appropriate care and follow-up, standards must exist both to assess all newborns prior to hospital discharge and to determine what interventions are necessary after this point. This manual offers standards by which nurse educators, nurse managers, nurse practitioners, nurses, physicians, home care providers, and insurers can assure universal access to needed services for all newborns. Not all newborns need an ongoing plan of support through home visiting. All newborns do, however, require universal access to risk assessment to determine the need for home visiting services.

Home visiting may be necessary due to psychosocial risk factors such as teen pregnancy or lack of prenatal care. Nationally, for infants born to mothers in these categories, morbidity and mortality occur at 2 to 3 times the incidence of that for infants born to mothers in other categories. We know these newborns have greater than average problems for which home visiting can provide better outcomes.

Some newborns born with psychosocial risk factors also present with physical risk factors such as drug dependency and low birthweight. Still other newborns born to mothers with no known psychosocial risk factors present with various physical problems. These can include prematurity, congenital anomaly, neurologic insults, and respiratory compromises.

■ DIRECTIONS FOR USE OF THE NEWBORN UNIVERSAL HOME RISK ASSESSMENT

1. The Newborn Universal Home Risk Assessment Procedure includes the following:

   a. Directions for use

   b. The Newborn Home Risk Assessment Tool

   c. Newborn Psychosocial Risk Assessment Standards

   d. Newborn Physical Risk Assessment Standards

2. A referral form should be completed by the source making the referral to the home health agency. Referrals for initial visits can be made by the physician, nurse practitioner, nurse, social worker, client, outreach, or another significant person involved in the newborn's care.

3. The agency, provider, and insurers will make all attempts to determine whether the mother or the newborn has had previous home care services in this pregnancy to assure appropriate coordination of care, access to medical history, and referral to the previous provider if appropriate.

4. The parent or guardian will be advised in advance of client rights in compliance with federal Medicare requirements.

5. All Plans of Care will be supervised by a physician in compliance with Medicare.

6. It is recommended that all newborns, especially those at or below the poverty level, be afforded access to the Universal Home Risk Assessment to determine the following:

   a. If there are risk factors that were not obvious during the prenatal period.

   b. If there are any plans for community services.

   c. If there is an ongoing need for home care services.

7. Based on the findings of this assessment, clients may be discharged from home care to their primary care provider or admitted to home care for follow-up based on short-term medical needs of the mother or infant.

8. Guidelines by risk category

   a. Initial assessment: All newborns will receive an initial home visit for physical and psychosocial assessment and determination of level of risk.

   b. Initial risk-specific home care

      1) Increased risk: All newborns determined to have one or more level 1 risk factors are eligible for one to three visits per month for 62 days, depending on individual need and per the physician's Plan of Care.

      2) Moderate risk: All newborns determined to have one or more level 2 risk factors are eligible for one to three visits per week for 62 days, depending on individual need and per the physician's Plan of Care.

      3) Maximal risk: All newborns determined to have one or more level 3 risk factors are eligible for four to seven visits per week for 62 days, depending on individual need and per the physician's Plan of Care.

   c. Ongoing risk-specific home care: The risk status of all newborns will be reassessed every 62 days and, depending on individual risk level and need, a new Plan of Care will be developed and implemented.

9. Newborns receiving the Newborn Universal Home Risk Assessment and meeting the following High-Risk Newborn Admission Criteria are admitted to the High-Risk Infant Follow-up Program.

   a. The infant's birth weight is 1500 grams or less.

   b. The mother is 17 years old or younger.

   c. There has been inadequate prenatal care.

   d. The mother or infant has tested positive in a urine drug screen (UDS) or has tested positive for alcohol or drug abuse.

   e. Mother or infant suffers from immunosuppression.

   f. Medical necessity dictates home care. The reason must be specified (i.e., Apgar at 5 minutes <5, respiratory distress syndrome [RDS; mechanical vent >6 hours], intracranial hemorrhage, major congenital anomalies, central nervous system (CNS) infection or trauma, hyperbilirubinemia [>25 mg/dl], neonatal seizures, gastroesophageal reflux, congenitally acquired infection or disease, intensive care nursery, or another medical or social necessity determined by the pediatric health care provider).

10. Any problems identified will be reported to the pediatric health care provider. A Plan of Care will be developed for newborns with the admission criteria listed above. Newborns not meeting the admission criteria will have a community service plan developed by the pediatric health care provider.

11. As part of the screening, the nurse will complete both the physical and psychosocial risk assessments to help identify client needs for services in the home and community. Newborn psychosocial risk assessment standards should be used to assure objectivity and to maximize use of services.

12. Levels of care
    After the initial evaluation, a Plan of Care will be developed in compliance with home health licensure and certification standards. The goals and objectives of the plan are based on the individual newborn's needs as identified by the screening.
    As part of the risk assessment section of the tool, the problems are assigned corresponding identifiers indicating a suggested level of care (i.e., a, cultural beliefs; b, inadequate food; c, current/recent abuse of drugs). These levels provide guidelines by which the agency, health care provider, client, and insurer can realistically plan for home care service need, directing the greatest intensity toward the greatest risks for poor outcome or preventable hospitalization. One rating (or more) in the next level qualifies the client for the higher level of care. For example, a client scoring all 1's would be at minimal risk, qualifying for level 1 services. If the client scored all 1's and a 2, that client would be at moderate risk and would therefore qualify for level 2 services.
    Initial plan guidelines include the following:

   a. Level 1: One to three visits per month for the first 62 days. If meeting high-risk admission criteria, the client will be reevaluated every 62 days through the infant's first year, unless discharged.

   b. Level 2: One to three visits per week for the first 62 days. If meeting high-risk admission criteria, the client will be reevaluated every 62 days through the infant's first year, unless discharged.

    c. Level 3: Four to seven visits per week for the first 62 days. If meeting high-risk admission criteria, the client will be reevaluated every 62 days through the infant's first year, unless discharged.

13. Newborns are discharged if the goals set for the infant are met or for one of the following reasons:

    a. There are no identified admission criteria justifying home care.

    b. The admission criterion problem has been identified and resolved at the initial visit.

    c. The goals in the established Plan of Care have been met.

    d. The goals cannot be met and the reasons are justified.

■ NEWBORN UNIVERSAL RISK ASSESSMENT: DEFINITIONS

PURPOSE: The purpose of this form is to provide the health professional with a screening tool to use in interviewing clients and to identify referral possibilities. The primary use of the form is in assessing risk and referring newborns at risk to appropriate services.

The key denotes priority referrals; however, in all cases, professional judgment must be used. Any factor or combination of factors could indicate a need for a referral if the professional performing the assessment thinks that the patient would benefit. Interdisciplinary cooperation should be assured.

1. Life transitions: Life events that result in the possibility of changes in lifestyle, perceptions, behaviors, or belief systems.

    a. Denial or rejection of pregnancy: *Denial* is defined on a cognitive and emotional level as not acknowledging/accepting the pregnancy. *Rejection* is defined as a strong negative emotional or behavioral response to being pregnant.

    b. Past/current/recent incest or rape victim: Any evidence of sexual abuse or assault (incest or rape).

    c. History of chronic disability: Any diagnosed chronic physical or mental disability.

    d. History of fetal death or other infant or pregnancy loss: Any loss that has occurred prenatally or within the infant's first year of life.

    e. Adoption or termination considered: Family seriously considering adoption or termination.

    f. Suspected domestic violence: Suspected battering of child, parent or guardian, or both. Possible law enforcement involvement.

2. Emotional status: Identifiable affect (demeanor, emotional tones), mental status (intellectual functions; use of defenses; orientation to place, person, time), or emotional status (emotional control, emotional appropriateness) of parent or guardian or significant other.

    a. History of mental illness, mental health treatment, or hospitalization: Diagnosis of mental illness that may have included outpatient treatment.

   b. Unresolved grief or significant loss: Inability to reach acceptance in dealing with significant losses such as death of significant other, loss of job or home, financial security, relationship with significant other, or divorce.

   c. Suicidal ideation: Serious suicidal tendencies as indicated by verbal threats, extreme depressed states, history of previous suicide attempts, and an actual suicide plan.

   d. Feelings of isolation, loneliness, or having inadequate support system: Expression of extreme loneliness. Parent or guardian may have family members or significant other present, but these people may provide insufficient or no emotional or financial support.

   e. Questionable coping: Difficulties in adjusting to and accepting social relationships, life opportunities, activities of daily living (ADLs), and self-concept.

   f. History of depression: Evidence of a debilitating depression (e.g., inability to take care of personal needs or even a single task, inability to bond or care for the child, potential abuse or neglect of self or others).

   g. Evidence of low self-esteem: Verbal or nonverbal expression of low self-esteem, evidenced by lack of eye contact, downgrading one's self, disheveled appearance, withdrawal, negative self-concept.

3. Substance abuse or risk-taking behavior: Ongoing use or abuse of substances and evidence of risky behavior (e.g., multiple sex partners, no birth control method, tobacco use, behavioral problems in general).

   a. Current or recent abuse of alcohol: Ongoing use or use within past year of alcohol as it impacts on the individual and family. Includes those with no recent abuse but still living with other abusers.

   b. Current or recent abuse of street drugs: Ongoing use or use within past year of illicit drugs (e.g., heroin, marijuana, cocaine, barbiturates, amphetamines) or a referral from a drug abuse program. History of use or continuing abuse as it impacts on the individual and family. Includes those with no recent abuse but still living with other abusers.

   c. Current or recent use or abuse of prescribed medication: Ongoing use or use within past year of prescribed medication as it impacts on the individual and family. Includes those with no recent abuse but still living with other abusers.

   d. Law enforcement involvement: Law enforcement involvement with regard to impact on the parent's ability to access care or to care for the child.

   e. Sexual risk-taking behaviors: Includes but is not limited to multiple sex partners, no method of birth control, and unsafe sex practices. Includes those who live in crack houses.

   f. Tobacco use or secondhand smoke exposure: Ongoing use of tobacco (cigarettes, chewing tobacco, snuff) by the child or family member and its impact on the risk of secondhand smoke exposure.

4. Parenting issues (observed or expressed): A parent's perception of himself or herself in the role of parent in relation to the actual behaviors that are observed or expressed by the client.

   a. Teenaged or inexperienced parents: The particular developmental stage of the parent and how it impacts the ability to parent or nurture the child. Examples: a child raising a child, or an inexperienced parent exhibiting lack of confidence and fears regarding the ability to meet the needs of the child.

   b. Developmental issues (child or family expectations): Lack of knowledge or poor understanding of what is age-appropriate for the developing child. Inappropriate expectations may lead to punitive responses. Example: expecting an 18-month-old to toilet train and then punishing the child if there are continued "accidents."

   c. Discipline issues: Discipline methods are often culturally learned behaviors. Problems can occur when discipline is not appropriate to the child's developmental stage. Example: disciplining a crying 3-month-old because the child is perceived as being bad and deliberately crying to upset the parents.

   d. Relationship issues (bonding or nurturing): Poor eye contact, coldness, mother unable to cuddle with child (which can lead to failure to thrive).

   e. History of child abuse or neglect, now resolved: History of placement of other children due to abuse or neglect, currently resolved.

   f. Child abuse or neglect, or current child protective service agency involvement:: Uncertainty regarding the possibility of abuse or neglect and anyone with current DHS involvement. The staff person who directly observes possible abuse or neglect is required by law to report this. Assure interdisciplinary involvement and follow-up.

   g. Three or more children younger than 6 years of age: The possibility of increased stress related to the care of multiple young children with little support or few social outlets.

5. Educational or cultural barriers: These are potential barriers that are associated with greater than average pediatric mortality and morbidity or that might impede the child's or the family's ability to follow instructions, meet expectations, or add to a recommended Plan of Care. Referrals might enhance the likelihood of appropriate use of services.

   a. Low literacy or limited intellectual ability: Evidence of inability or difficulty in reading basic instructions. Documentation of low or borderline intellectual capabilities.

   b. Language barriers: Inability to communicate basic information in English; also includes hearing and speech impairments.

   c. Cognitive deficits: Documented or perceived deficits in the ability to process information.

   d. Parent or guardian has not completed school beyond grade 12.

   e. Parent or guardian has not completed school beyond grade 10.

   f. Parent or guardian has not completed school beyond grade 9.

   g. Culture or beliefs: Cultural factors and beliefs that may impact health attitudes and behaviors, such as religious beliefs and practices, health values, attitudes toward getting and receiving health care, and present behaviors and lifestyle. These factors will vary among communities and individuals, and providers should be prepared to identify and respond to the needs of the populations they serve. Examples: cereal in an infant's bottle, jewelry for the baby, socks to cure hiccups, and coffee grounds to treat conjunctivitis.

6. Economic or resource needs: These factors could be appropriately handled through case management or, if more than one factor presents significant stress, through psychosocial intervention.

   a. Insufficient income or no income to meet basic needs.

   b. No transportation: Inability to secure adequate transportation to meet instrumental ADLs. This may include a child or family member's inability to plan or to take responsibility for required decision-making.

   c. Inadequate food: Difficulty in obtaining food to meet basic nutritional needs. May include lack of resources to purchase food or lack of knowledge about available resources.

   d. Legal needs: Need for assistance from the legal system (e.g., pediatric support, divorce, domestic violence). May include lack of resources to secure legal aid or empowerment to effectively access available legal resources.

   e. Chronic difficulty accessing system: Persistent inability to access multiple agencies to assist with resources, impairing the ability to meet the most basic needs.

   f. Pediatric care problems: Problems securing adequate acceptable pediatric care such that gaining employment or accessing medical care is difficult or of low priority.

   g. Medicaid or general medical insurance problems: No existing permanent medical coverage for medical condition.

7. Infant medical or nutritional factors

   a. Abnormal physical findings on this assessment: Any abnormal findings as noted in item 1 of the Newborn Home Risk Assessment Tool.

   b. Prenatal exposure to drugs or alcohol: Maternal use of drugs and/or alcohol during pregnancy.

   c. Infant anemia: hemoglobin <14.5 for a newborn, <9 for a 2-month-old, <11.5 for a 6- to 12-year-old.

   d. Failure to thrive in siblings, previous or existing: Suspected or medically diagnosed and documented history and/or current condition.

   e. Diagnosed or suspected malabsorption: Suspected or medically diagnosed and documented disorders (e.g., inadequate absorption of nutrients caused by one or combination of the following: infections, routine enteropathy, pancreatic insufficiency, gastric resection, antibiotic therapy, etc.).

   f. Symptoms of intolerance to formula: A child with overt symptoms of formula intolerance may present with any or all of these problems:

      1) Diarrhea (watery, large, frequent bowel movements that have a bad odor)

      2) Vomiting (throwing up large amounts of the stomach contents through the mouth)

      3) Constipation (painful bowel movements that are difficult to pass and look like small, hard balls)

      4) Abdominal distention

      5) Rash

      6) Bloody stools

      7) Other babies may present with milder symptoms similar to those of overt formula intolerance:

         (a) Spitting up

         (b) Gas

         (c) Fussiness

   g. Gastroesophageal (GE) reflux: Medically diagnosed and documented GE reflux.

   h. Low birth weight infant: Weight less than 2500 grams at birth.

   i. Very low birth weight infant: Weight less than 1500 grams at birth.

   j. Inadequate prenatal care: Less than four prenatal visits, for any reason.

   k. Previous hospitalization of siblings in first year.

l. Extended neonatal intensive care unit (NICU) hospitalization: Neonatal course for the child that includes treatment and more than an overnight stay for observation in the NICU.

m. Medical problems related to prematurity: Any medical problem, current or residual, as a result of birth at or before 37 weeks.

n. Medical problems related to congenital anomalies: Any medical problem, current or residual, as a result of any congenital anomaly.

o. Sexually transmitted disease (STD) exposure in pregnancy, untreated: Documented STD, untreated or treatment not completed. Includes chlamydia, herpes, syphilis, gonorrhea, human immunodeficiency virus (HIV), and hepatitis.

p. Lead exposure: An answer of "yes" to any of the following risk-assessment questions means the child is at risk:

   1) Does your child live in or regularly visit a house built before 1960? Is/was your child's day care center/preschool/home built before 1960? Do any of these dwellings have peeling or chipping paint?

   2) Does your child live in a house built before 1960 with recent, ongoing, or planned renovation or remodeling?

   3) Have any of your children or their playmates had lead poisoning?

   4) Does your child frequently come in contact with an adult who works with lead? Examples are construction, welding, pottery, or other trades practiced in your community.

   5) Does you child live near a lead smelter, battery recycling plant, or other industry likely to release lead into the community? Cite other examples.

   6) Do you give your child any home or folk remedies that may contain lead?

   7) Does your child live near a heavily traveled major highway where soil or dust may be contaminated with lead?

   8) Does your home's plumbing have lead pipes or copper with lead solder joints?

8. Environmental problems

   a. Housing problems: Includes any of the following:

      1) Living space or accommodations inadequate for the number of occupants in the household, indicating that a potential health or safety hazard exists.

      2) Conditions that are substandard, indicating that clear safety hazards exist (e.g., poor sanitation, ventilation, heating, electrical hazards, vector infestation).

      3) Movement from one house/apartment/shelter to another without a stable home base or a network of support systems. This could include the migrant population.

      4) Without housing, totally reliant on community support for shelter, or living on the streets.

   b. Utilities: Lack of electricity, heat, phone, or air conditioning in those situations where they are basic necessities.

   c. Water/sewer: Lack of water/sewer.

   d. Refrigeration: Lack of refrigeration.

   e. Unsafe neighborhood: Neighborhood is an area of high crime or otherwise known to be unsafe for its residents. This would include a known drug area.

f. Inadequate preparation for infant: Lack of preparation for meeting the basic needs of a newborn in the home (e.g., no crib, car seat, clothing, formula).

▨ STANDARDS OF CARE FOR INFANT ASSESSMENT

1. Skin

    a. *Standards within normal limits (WNL):* Skin color should be pink and the skin should be warm to touch; some mottling may be present in extremities. A slightly yellow color with blanching about nose or the presence of a normal newborn rash, birthmark, or mongolian spots is also a normal finding.

    b. *Deviations:* Evidence of cyanosis about face or lips requires investigation; the infant who appears very pale or ruddy should be evaluated. Icterus, a yellow skin tone to blanching about face and abdomen, is also an abnormal finding. Another finding to investigate is a rash appearing to be spreading out from inside the anus. Any rash characterized by bright red papules that may erupt and form craterlike ulcers or that appears to contain pustules is cause for further assessment.

    c. *Evaluation of deviations:* Observe the degree of cyanosis while the infant is eating or crying. Evaluate the activity level, vital signs, heart and lung sounds, effect of posturing infant, suck, interest and ability to maintain time needed to feed. If there is evidence of icterus, determine if bilirubin was drawn in the hospital and if the mother had instructions for follow-up. Determine, if possible, the mother's and infant's blood types. (If the mother is type O, determine if she received RhoGAM; report immediately to the health care provider if the baby has a positive blood type and the mother did not receive RhoGAM). Evaluate the infant's activity level, interest in feeds, color of stools, and the presence of yellow in sclera. If the baby has a suspicious rash, evaluate the maternal history of infection and the length of time from rupture of membrane (ROM). Assess other vital signs and check for signs and symptoms of infection in the infant. Determine if the baby's health care provider is aware of the rash and what treatment has been prescribed.

    d. *Action:* If infant's skin tone is yellow to blanching about abdomen or if sclera appears yellow, assess the infant and notify the health care provider from the client's home. If the infant is slightly yellow only about the face, is active, alert, and eating well, instruct the mother to provide extra water after feeds and with signs and symptoms of jaundice (yellow about abdomen or sclera, lethargy, decreased interest in feeds). The family should be aware to notify the health care provider if the signs and symptoms increase. If the infant has a rash and is not under the health care provider's care, notify the health care provider of your findings from the client's home.

2. Head

    a. *Standards WNL:* A rounded head is normal; some molding may be apparent. Axillary temperature should be between 97°F and 99°F.

    b. *Deviations:* Caput succedaneum, which may cross cranial sutures, merits further evaluation. Cephalhematoma, which does not cross cranial sutures, is also an abnormal finding. If the infant is unable to move his or her head from side to side, it may indicate neurologic trauma. Asymmetrical flattened occiput on either side of head may indicate plagiocephaly. If the infant holds his or her head at an angle, torticollis is a possibility. An axillary temperature below 97°F or above 99°F, or swings of more than 2°F from one reading to the next are also abnormal findings.

   c. *Evaluation of deviations:* If you suspect caput succedaneum or cephalhematoma, evaluate the infant's neurologic reflexes. Evaluate for signs and symptoms of intracranial hemorrhage (abnormal respiration with cyanosis, shrill cry, reduced responsiveness, tense fontanelle, and convulsions—twitching of the lower jaw with salivation is often a sign of convulsion). If head movement, asymmetrical flattened occiput, or the head's angle is a problem, instruct the parents to change the infant's sleeping positions frequently and call the health care provider if there is no improvement.

      For temperature problems, keep in mind that infant temperature may rise to 100.2°F or decrease to 96.6°F if the infant is exposed to excessive warmth or chill. The infant should be wrapped or unwrapped according to temperature deviation. Retake the child's temperature in 15 minutes. Evaluate the infant for signs and symptoms of sepsis or other infection (poor suck, anorexia, regurgitation of feeds, diarrhea, jaundice, pallor, cyanosis, tremors, lethargy, hyper- or hyporeflexes, bradypnea, petechiae). Review the maternal history of infections and length of time ROM. Teach the parents to use a thermometer. Assess their ability to read the thermometer.

   d. *Action:* Educate the parents that caput and cephalhematoma will resolve. Contact the health care provider if signs or symptoms of intracranial hemorrhage or neurologic problems are suspected. If head movement, asymmetrical flattened occiput, or the head's angle is a problem, document the condition for the health care provider to review at the first well-baby visit. For the infant with a temperature, if a rise and fall of temperature does not occur and the infant is free of signs and symptoms of infection and other vital signs are WNL, the mother should retake the child's temperature in 1 hour and call the health care provider if there is no improvement. If signs and symptoms of sepsis or any type of infection are present, the nurse must call the health care provider from the client's home. If the child's temperature is below 96.6°F or above 100.2°F, call the health care provider immediately. Call the health care provider if the child's temperature swings 2°F or more from one reading to next.

3. Neck

   a. *Standards WNL:* Short, straight creases with skin folds are normal. The posterior neck lacks loose extra folds of skin. The head should move freely from side to side.

   b. *Deviations:* An abnormally short neck is cause for further investigation. The following conditions also require attention: arching or inability to flex the neck (meningitis, congenital anomaly, webbing of neck, Turner's syndrome, Down's syndrome, trisomy 18) and neck rigidity (congenital torticollis, 11th nerve damage).

   c. *Evaluation of deviations:* Collect more data indicative of chromosomal aberrations. Determine the maternal history of infections and length of time from rupture of membrane. Assess the infant for signs of infection.

   d. *Action:* If a congenital defect is suspected, contact the health care provider and the agency for consultation outside of the client's home. If the infant evidences signs or symptoms of infection, contact the health care provider from the client's home.

4. Eyes

   a. *Standards WNL:* The cornea and retina should be clear. The ability to follow a light with the eyes is notable.

   b. *Deviations:* Ulceration (herpes infection), large cornea or corneas of unequal size (congenital glaucoma), or clouding, opacity of lens (cataract) are all abnormal findings.

   c. *Evaluation of deviations:* Determine the history of maternal infection and the length of time ROM. Determine if the health care provider is aware of deviation.

    d. *Action:* Contact the health care provider from the client's home unless the mother indicates that the baby is already under treatment by the health care provider for the deviation.

5. Pupils

    a. *Standards WNL:* The pupils should be equal in size and round, and should react to light by accommodation.

    b. *Deviations:* Abnormal findings include unequal pupils (CNS damage), dilatation or constriction (intracranial damage, retinoblastoma, glaucoma), and pupils that are nonreactive to light or accommodation (brain injury).

    c. *Evaluation of deviations:* Assess neurologic reflexes.

    d. *Action:* Report your findings to the baby's health care provider from the client's home.

6. Conjunctiva

    a. *Standards WNL:* Chemical conjunctivitis (subsides in 2 to 7 days), palpebral conjunctiva (red, not hyperemic), and subconjunctival hemorrhage are all within normal limits.

    b. *Deviations:* The following conditions are not within normal limits: pale color (anemia), inflammation or edema, purulent drainage (infection, blocked tear duct).

    c. *Evaluation of deviations:* Determine the history of maternal infections and the length of time ROM. Determine the history of eye drainage and if under treatment by a health care provider for deviation.

    d. *Action:* Contact the health care provider from the client's home if the baby is not under treatment for the deviation.

7. Eyes/vision

    a. *Standards WNL:* The infant should be able to track moving object to midline. The ability to follow a light with the eyes is notable.

    b. *Deviations:* Cataracts (congenital) or infections are abnormal findings.

    c. *Evaluation of deviations:* Determine the history of maternal infections during pregnancy.

    d. *Action:* Record any questions about visual activity for the health care provider to follow-up at the first well-baby check-up.

8. General appearance

    a. *Standards WNL:* Eyes should be bright and clear, evenly placed, with slight nystagmus, concomitant strabismus, and should move in all directions. At birth, eyes are blue-slate in color, or brown in babies of color.

    b. *Deviations:* Gross nystagmus (damage to the third, fourth, and sixth cranial nerves), constant and fixed strabismus, lack of pigmentation (albinism), and Brushfield's spots (may indicate Down's syndrome) are all abnormal findings. "Sunset eyes," ptosis, and an upward slant in nonorientals should be investigated as well.

    c. *Evaluation of deviations:* Determine what information was given to the mother in the hospital. Do not upset the family with only suspected defects. Call the health care provider and the agency for consultation from your home prior to presenting your suspicions to family. Evaluate neurologic status.

    d. *Action:* Indicate to the parent that you will call your report in to the health care provider. Call the health care provider and the agency from your home. Follow the instructions of the health care provider and the agency.

9. Ears

   a. *Standards WNL:* Ears should be well formed. They may have minor anomalies such as auricular fistulas and tubercles. A twisted or rotated ear may give the false impression of being low set.

   b. *Deviations:* Gross malformations or low-set ears are not within normal limits.

   c. *Evaluation of deviations:* Evaluate the setting of the ears by holding a pen or pencil from the outer canthus of the eye. This should give a straight appearance, as if wearing glasses.

   d. *Action:* Identify with the parent if the health care provider is aware of the deviation. Report to the physician from the client's home if the parent states that the health care provider is unaware of the deviation.

10. Nose/external nasal aspects

    a. *Standards WNL:* The nose may appear flattened as a result of delivery process. Patent nares bilaterally.

    b. *Deviations:* A continued flat or broad bulge of nose (Down's syndrome) or blockage of the nares (mucus or secretions) is abnormal.

    c. *Evaluation of deviations:* Assess for signs and symptoms of infection.

    d. *Action:* Consult with physician from your home if you suspect a congenital defect. If signs and symptoms of infection are present, contact the health care provider from the client's home. If there are no signs and symptoms of infection, instruct in the use of a bulb syringe if available. The family should contact the health care provider if the problem persists.

11. Nose/internal aspects

    a. *Standards WNL:* Pink and firm mucous membranes are within normal limits. The septum should be midline and without polyps or tumors.

    b. *Deviations:* A deviated or perforated septum, or tumors or polyps of the septum are abnormal findings. Swelling and erythema also are notable.

    c. *Evaluation of deviations:* Determine the infant's ability to make good air exchange, auscultate lungs, and assess restlessness and irritability. Assess for signs and symptoms of infection or distress.

    d. *Action:* Determine if the baby's health care provider is following a deviation. Contact the provider from the client's home if the infant appears to experience any distress.

12. Mouth/function of facial, hypoglossopharyngeal, and vagus nerves

    a. *Standards WNL:* Symmetry of movement and strength are normal findings. Assess for adequate salivation, presence of gag, swallowing, and sucking reflexes. The tongue should be midline.

    b. *Deviations:* If the mouth draws to one side, it may indicate transient seventh cranial nerve paralysis due to pressure in utero or trauma during delivery or congenital paralysis. A fishlike shape may indicate Treacher Collins syndrome. Suppressed or absent reflexes are also abnormal. Deviations from midline could imply cranial nerve damage.

    c. *Evaluation of deviations:* Evaluate other neurologic functions.

    d. *Action:* Notify the health care provider from the client's home if the parent states that the provider is unaware of the deviation.

13. Palate (soft and hard)

   a. *Standards WNL:* The hard palate should be dome shaped and the uvula should be midline with symmetric movement of the soft palate. The palate should be intact, and the infant should suck well when stimulated. Epithelial (Epstein's) pearls often appear on mucosa.

   b. *Deviations:* A high-steepled palate could be a sign of Treacher Collins syndrome. Clefts in either the hard or soft palate may point to a polygenic disorder.

   c. *Evaluation of deviations:* Evaluate infant hydration, ability to feed, respiratory status, and parental bonding.

   d. *Action:* The infant with a cleft palate will be under a health care provider's care. Report the progress of the baby to the health care provider from the client's home.

14. Pharynx

   a. *Standards WNL:* The pharynx should be unobstructed, with no drainage in the back of the throat and no exudate on the tonsils. The esophagus should be patent; some drooling is common in newborns.

   b. *Deviations:* If exudate is present, it may be a sign of infection. Excessive drooling or bubbling may point to esophageal atresia.

   c. *Evaluation of deviations:* If exudate is present, examine for other signs of infection. For possible esophageal atresia, evaluate possible esophageal defects by reviewing the infant's feeding history.

   d. *Action:* Report all abnormal findings to the health care provider from the client' s home.

15. Tongue

   a. *Standards WNL:* The tongue should be free-moving in all directions and midline. It should have a pink color, with a smooth to rough texture, noncoated. The tongue should also be proportional to the mouth. Sucking and rooting reflexes should be present. The infant should be able to discriminate pleasant from unpleasant tastes.

   b. *Deviations:* The following are not within normal limits: Lack of movement or asymmetric movement, tongue-tied; white cheesy coating (thrush); deep ridges; a large tongue with short frenulum (cretinism, Down's and other mental retardation syndromes); and absence of reaction of tongue to various stimuli (seventh cranial nerve damage).

   c. *Evaluation of deviations:* If there is a lack of movement, further assess neurologic functions. Test reflexes, elevation of tongue when depressed with tongue blade. Check for signs of weakness or deviation. If there is a white coating, differentiate between thrush and milk curds. Reassure the parents that the tongue pattern may change from day to day. For all other deviations, evaluate neurologic status and assess neurologic functions.

   d. *Action:* Notify the health care provider from the client's home if a deviation or infection is suspected. Consult with the health care provider from your home whenever a congenital defect is suspected.

16. Gums

   a. *Standards WNL:* The gums should be dark pink, firm, and smooth. There will be a dark (melanotic) line along the gums in black babies.

   b. *Deviations:* Inflamed gums (infection), pallor (anemia), and precocious teeth should all be examined more closely.

   c. *Evaluation of deviations:* Evaluate for other signs and symptoms of anemia or infection.

   d. *Action:* Notify the health care provider from the client's home if anemia or infection is suspected.

17. Lips

    a. *Standards WNL:* Labial tubercle (pink, sucking blisters) is normal. Mucosa of lips should be well demarcated from the surrounding skin. Saliva should be scant. Lips fused in midline.

    b. *Deviations:* Cleft lip (polygenic disorder) and a thin upper lip require closer inspection.

    c. *Evaluation of deviations:* Counsel parents on special feeding techniques that may be necessary if the child has a cleft lip. Assess for fetal alcohol syndrome if the child has a thin upper lip.

    d. *Action:* For a cleft lip, parents should be aware to contact the health care provider if feeding problems persist. If the child has fetal alcohol syndrome, refer the family to an early intervention program.

18. Chest/clavicles

    a. *Standards WNL:* The clavicles should be straight and intact, the moro reflex should be elicitable, and there should be bilateral movement of both shoulders.

    b. *Deviations:* The following conditions require further examination: a knot or lump on clavicle (fracture during difficult delivery), or a unilateral moro reflex response on unaffected side (fracture of clavicle, brachial palsy, Erb–Duchenne syndrome).

    c. *Evaluation of deviations:* For a knot or lump on the clavicle, obtain a detailed labor and delivery history. Assess respiratory status.

    d. *Action:* Notify the health care provider from the client's home if a deviation is suspected that is not already diagnosed and under treatment.

19. Appearance and size of chest

    a. *Standards WNL:* The circumference should be 32.5 cm or 1 to 2 cm less than the head. The chest should be wider than it is long; it should be of a normal shape without depressed or prominent sternum. The lower end of the sternum (xiphoid cartilage) may be protruding; this is less apparent after several weeks. The sternum should be about 8 cm long.

    b. *Deviations:* Funnel chest (congenital or associated with Marfan's syndrome), continued protrusion of xiphoid cartilage (Marfan's syndrome; "pigeon chest"), and barrel chest are findings beyond normal limits.

    c. *Evaluation of deviations:* If Marfan's syndrome is suspected, measure at the level of the nipples after exhalation. For barrel chest, determine the adequacy of other respiratory and circulatory signs. Assess for other signs and symptoms of various syndromes.

    d. *Action:* Notify the health care provider from the client's home if a deviation is suspected or apparent.

20. Expansion and retraction

    a. *Standards WNL:* Bilateral expansion or no intracostal, subcostal, or suprasternal retraction are normal findings.

    b. *Deviations:* Unequal chest expansion (pneumonia, pneumothorax respiratory distress) and retractions (respiratory distress) are abnormal findings.

    c. *Evaluation of deviations:* Collect more data regarding respiratory effort if chest expansion is unequal (regulatory, flaring of nares, difficulty on both inspiration and expiration). If there are retractions, examine the chest thoroughly using the techniques of inspection, palpation, and auscultation.

    d. *Action:* Notify the health care provider from the client's home if a deviation is suspected or apparent.

21. Chest percussion

    a. *Standards WNL:* Decreased percussion over liver, diaphragm, and heart, with these areas well demarcated, is within normal limits.

    b. *Deviations:* Dullness in lung fields (consolidation of lungs, atelectasis) or hyperresonance of the chest (pneumonia, pneumothorax, distended stomach) should be evaluated further.

    c. *Evaluation of deviations:* Examine the chest thoroughly using the techniques of inspection, palpation, and auscultation.

    d. *Action:* Notify the health care provider from the client's home if a deviation is suspected or apparent.

22. Auscultation

    a. *Standards WNL:* Breath sounds are louder in infants and heard bilaterally. The chest and axilla clear on crying.

    b *Deviations:* Decreased breath sounds may indicate decreased respiratory activity, atelectasis, pneumothorax. Increased breath sounds are heard with resolving pneumonia.

    c. *Evaluation of deviations:* Perform a complete physical exam and collaborate with the health care provider regarding positive findings.

    d. *Action:* Notify the health care provider from the client's home if a deviation is suspected or apparent.

23. Respiratory rate

    a. *Standards WNL:* The respiratory rate should be between 30 to 60 breaths per minute.

    b. *Deviations:* A rate below 30 and above 60 requires follow up.

    c. *Evaluation of deviations:* Assess the infant's entire respiratory status and observe color and activity level to determine adequate oxygenation. The infant with a respiratory rate between 20 and 30 breaths per minute may be receiving adequate oxygenation; the rate should increase with stimulation. A rate from 60 to 80 without other signs of distress may be due to increased activity (crying, etc.). Assess and collaborate with the health care provider if questionable.

    d. *Action:* Notify the health care provider from the client's home of a rate below 20/min or above 80/min, or if any signs or symptoms of distress are noted, regardless of rate.

24. Bronchial breath sounds (heard when trachea and bronchi closest to chest wall, above sternum and between scapulae) and determination of point of maximal impulse (PMI)

    a. *Standards WNL:* Bronchial sounds bilaterally. The air entry is clear. Rates may indicate normal newborn atelectasis. Cough reflex absent at birth, appears in 2 or more days. It is difficult to assess exact PMI in an infant under 2 years old, but usually at lateral to midclavicular line at third or fourth interspace.

    b. *Deviations:* Adventitious or abnormal sounds (respiratory diseases or distress) and malpositioning (enlargement, abnormal placement, pneumothorax, dextrocardia, diaphragmatic hernia) require investigation.

    c. *Evaluation of deviations:* Initiate cardiac and respiratory evaluation.

    d. *Action:* Notify the health care provider from the client's home of any suspected deviation.

25. Breasts

    a. *Standards WNL:* Breasts should be flat with symmetrical nipple. Breast tissue has a diameter of 5 cm or more at term. The distance between nipples is 8 cm. Breast engorgement occurs on the third day of life, and liquid discharge may be expressed in term infants.

    b. *Deviations:* A lack of breast tissue may indicate prematurity or SGA (small for gestational age). Breast abscesses are not within the normal limits.

    c. *Evaluation of deviations:* Reassure parents that breast engorgement is normal. Assess for signs and symptoms of infection.

    d. *Action:* Notify the health care provider from the client's home of any deviations present or if a follow-up appointment is required sooner than the normal well-baby follow up, due to SGA, prematurity, or low birth weight.

26. Heart auscultation and palpation

    a. *Standards WNL:* The heart lies horizontally, with the left border extending to the left of midclavicle. There should be a regular rhythm and rate. Functional murmurs may be present, no thrills, with a split second sound (lub, splat). Heart rate should be 100 to 160.

    b. *Deviations:* Arrhythmia (anoxia), tachycardia, bradycardia are abnormal findings. Location of murmurs (possible congenital cardiac anomaly) also requires further study. Rates between 90 to 100 and 160 to 180 require evaluation for adequate oxygenation, good circulatory effort, increase or decrease with corresponding activity level. Respiratory rate should be within normal limits. Rates at 90 (sleeping) or at 180 (crying).

    c. *Evaluation of deviations:* Evaluate any murmur: location, timing, and duration; observe for accompanying cardiac pathology symptoms, and ascertain any family history.

    d. *Action:* All arrhythmia and gallop rhythms should be referred to the health care provider from the client's home. Report any evidence of circulatory compromise. Report to the health care provider any rate below 90 or above 180, even if the infant appears to be in no distress.

27. Trachea (palpate from top to bottom with thumb and index fingers)

    a. *Standards WNL:* The trachea should be slightly right of midline.

    b. *Deviations:* Deviated left or right (pneumothorax, tumor of chest or neck) is not within normal limits.

    c. *Evaluation of deviations:* Initiate cardiopulmonary evaluation.

    d. *Action:* Notify the health care provider from the client's home if a deviation is suspected.

28. Rib cage and diaphragm

    a. *Standards WNL:* A horizontal groove at the diaphragm shows flaring of the rib cage to a mild degree.

    b. *Deviations:* Harrison's groove with marked flaring indicates a vitamin D deficiency. Inadequacy of respiration movement requires further inquiry.

    c. *Evaluation of deviations:* Initiate cardiopulmonary evaluation.

    d. *Action:* Notify the health care provider from the client's home if a deviation is suspected.

29. Abdomen/appearance

    a. *Standards WNL:* The abdomen should be cylindrical with some protrusion and appear large in relation to pelvis; some laxness of abdominal muscles is normal. There should be no cyanosis and few vessels can be seen. Diastasis recti is common in black infants. Observe for synchronous movement with breathing.

    b. *Deviations:* A distended, shiny abdomen with engorged vessels may indicate gastrointestinal abnormalities, infection, or congenital megacolon. A scaphoid appearance may be evidence of a diaphragmatic hernia. Increased or decreased peristalsis needs to be evaluated. Localized flank bulging (enlarged kidneys, ascites, or absent abdominal muscles) also requires evaluation.

    c. *Evaluation of deviations:* Examine abdomen thoroughly for mass or organomegaly. For localized flank bulging, assess for other signs and symptoms of obstruction.

    d. Notify the health care provider from the client's home if a deviation is suspected or apparent.

30. Palpation

    a. *Standards WNL:* The abdomen should be nontender with no palpable masses.

    b. *Deviations:* A tense abdomen with marked rigidity or resistance to pressure may indicate infection. Solid mass (Wilms' tumor) or teratoma mass located below the umbilicus is abnormal finding.

    c. *Evaluation of deviations:* Take temperature and assess other signs and symptoms.

    d. *Action:* Notify the health care provider from the client's home if a deviation is suspected or apparent.

31. Umbilicus

    a. *Standards WNL:* There should be no protrusion of umbilicus and no umbilical hernia; protrusion of umbilicus is common in black infants. Umbilicus should be a bluish white color. Cutis navel (umbilical cord project) and granulation tissue in navel are normal. Two arteries and one vein should be apparent. It begins drying 1 to 2 hours after birth, blackens by 3 to 5 days, sloughs off by 7 to 9 days. There should be no bleeding.

    b. *Deviations:* The following conditions are abnormal findings: umbilical hernia, patent urachus (congenital malformation), omphalocele (congenital hernia), gastroschisis, redness or exudate around cord (infection), yellow discoloration (hemolytic disease, meconium staining), and a single umbilical artery (congenital anomalies).

    c. *Evaluation of deviations:* Measure an umbilical hernia by palpating the opening and record. It should close by 1 year of age. Instruct the parents on cord care and hygiene.

    d. *Action:* Notify the health care provider from the client's home if a deviation is suspected or apparent.

32. Liver

    a. *Standard WNL:* The liver should be 1 to 2 cm below the right costal margin.

    b. *Deviations:* An enlarged liver (sepsis, erythroblastosis) requires further evaluation.

    c. *Evaluation of deviations:* Note and record size, consistency, and tenderness.

    d. *Action:* Notify the health care provider from the client's home if a deviation is suspected or apparent.

33. Spleen

    a. *Standards WNL:* The tip should be under the left costal margin. Posterior flank should be firm, oval mass, not enlarged, less commonly palpable.

    b. *Deviations:* Enlarged spleen (trauma) or displaced kidney (Wilms' tumor, neuroblastoma, polycryptic kidney, agenesis) are not within normal limits.

    c. *Evaluation of deviations:* Assess hydration, voids, other signs and symptoms of infection, kidney failure.

    d. *Action:* Notify the health care provider from the client's home if a deviation is suspected or apparent.

34. Auscultation and percussion

    a. *Standards WNL:* Soft bowel sounds may be heard shortly after birth, every 10 to 30 seconds. Normal peristalsis. The abdomen has a tympanic sound except over the liver and spleen (dull sound).

    b. *Deviations:* Bowel sounds in chest (diaphragmatic hernia), an absence of bowel sounds, or hyperperistalsis (intestinal obstruction) are all abnormal findings. Increased dull sound (mass or organomegaly) also is abnormal.

    c. *Evaluation of deviations:* Assess respiratory status; history of bowel movement. Assess for other signs of dehydration or infection. Examine the abdomen thoroughly by light and deep palpation.

    d. *Action:* Notify the health care provider of suspicion and assessment from the client's home.

35. Femoral pulses

    a. *Standards WNL:* Femoral pulses should be palpable, equal, and bilateral.

    b. *Deviations:* Absent or diminished femoral pulses (coarctation of aorta) are not within normal limits.

    c. *Evaluation of deviations:* Evaluate cardiopulmonary status.

    d. *Action:* Notify the health care provider of suspicion and assessment from the client's home.

36. Inguinal area

    a. *Standards WNL:* There should be no bulges along inguinal area and no inguinal lymph nodes felt.

    b. *Deviations:* Inguinal hernia.

    c. *Evaluation of deviations:* Determine if the health care provider is aware of the deviation. Future instruction may be necessary.

    d. *Action:* Call the health care provider with your findings from the client's home unless the parent indicates the provider is already aware of the deviation.

37. Bladder

    a. *Standards WNL:* The bladder percusses 1 to 4 cm above symphysis pubis. It will be emptied about 3 hours after birth, if not at the time of birth. Urine is nonoffensive, with a mild odor.

    b. *Deviations:* Foul odor (infection) and failure to void within 24 hours after birth should be investigated.

   c. *Evaluation of deviations:* Assess hydration, common signs and symptoms of infection, and feeding history.

   d. *Action:* Notify the health care provider from the client's home to report the deviation.

38. Genitals

   a. *Standards WNL:* Gender should be clearly delineated.

   b. *Deviations:* Ambiguous genitals are an abnormal finding.

   c. *Evaluation of deviations:* Review the birth history and the follow-up plan of health care provider.

   d. *Action:* Call the health care provider from the client's home if no follow-up plan has been implemented.

39. Male penis

   a. *Standards WNL:* The penis should be slender in appearance, 2.5 cm long, 1 cm wide at birth. The normal urinary orifice, the urethral meatus, is at the tip of the penis. The urethral opening should be noninflamed. The foreskin adheres to glans, and prepuce can be retracted beyond the urethral opening. Uncircumcised foreskin should be tight after 2 to 3 months. Circumcised. Erectile tissue present.

   b. *Deviations:* Micropenis (congenital anomaly); meatal atresia, hypospadius, epispadius; urethritis (infection); ulceration of meatal opening, infection, inflammation; phimosis, if still tight after 3 months; no foreskin remaining on penis after circumcision are all abnormal findings.

   c. *Evaluation of deviations:* For meatal atresia, observe and record voiding history. For urethritis, palpate for enlarged inguinal lymph nodes and record painful micturition. If meatal opening is ulcerated, evaluate whether the ulcer is due to diaper rash or not. Counsel regarding care. Assess for signs and symptoms of infection. In cases of circumcision, teach parents how to care for circumcision. Teach parents not to retract foreskin of uncircumcised male until told to by health care provider.

   d. *Action:* Report any deviations to the health care provider. Collaborate with the health care provider in the presence of an abnormality.

40. Scrotum

   a. *Standards WNL:* Skin will be loose and hanging or tight and small, and extensive rugae will be present. Scrotum should be of normal size. Scrotal discoloration is common in breech. Skin should be a normal skin color.

   b. *Deviations:* Large scrotum containing fluid (hydrocele) and red, shiny scrotal skin (orchitis) are abnormal findings.

   c. *Evaluation of deviations:* For hydrocele, shine a light through scrotum (transilluminate) to verify diagnosis. For orchitis, assess for blood supply and tenderness or pain.

   d. *Action:* Notify the health care provider from the client's home of any suspected deviation or problem.

41. Testes

   a. *Standards WNL:* Testes will be descended at birth, and are not consistently found in scrotum. Testes should be 1.5 to 2 cm at birth.

   b. *Deviations:* Undescended testes (cryptorchidism), enlarged testes (tumor), and small testes (Klinefelter's syndrome or adrenal hyperplasia) require further examination.

   c. *Evaluation of deviations:* For cryptorchidism, if the testes cannot be felt in the scrotum, gently palpate femoral inguinal, perineal, and abdominal areas for presence.

   d. *Action:* Notify the health care provider from the client's home of any suspected deviation. Refer and collaborate with the health care provider for further diagnostic studies.

42. Female mons

   a. *Standards WNL:* The female mons should be a normal skin color. The area is pigmented in dark-skinned races. Labia majora cover labia minora, symmetrical size appropriate for gestational age.

   b. *Deviations:* Hematoma and lesions are abnormalities.

   c. *Evaluation of deviations:* Evaluate recent trauma.

   d. *Action:* Notify the health care provider from the client's home of any suspected deviation.

43. Clitoris

   a. *Standard WNL:* The clitoris is normally large in a newborn. Edema and bruising may occur in a breech delivery.

   b. *Deviations:* Hypertrophy (in size; hermaphrodism) is not within normal limits.

   c. *Evaluation of deviations:* Determine if the health care provider is aware of the deviation.

   d. *Action:* Notify the health care provider of your findings.

44. Vagina

   a. *Standards WNL:* Urinary meatus and vaginal orifice are visible (0.5 cm circumference). Vaginal tag or hymenal tag is present, which disappears in a few weeks. There may also be discharge or smegma under labia. Bloody or mucoid discharge is normal as well.

   b. *Deviations:* Inflammation, erythema, and discharge may indicate urethritis. Congenital absence of vagina is another possible problem. A foul-smelling discharge could mean infection. Excessive vaginal bleeding requires evaluation.

   c. *Evaluation of deviations:* If urethritis is suspected, assess for signs and symptoms of infection. Refer any congenital defects to the health care provider. If a discharge is present, collect data and further evaluate the reason for the discharge.

   d. *Action:* Notify the health care provider from the client's home of any suspected deviation.

CHAPTER 3

Standard Program for High-Risk Newborn Home Visiting Follow-Up

This program was developed after 6 years of research in problems related to newborn mortality. The home health agency that developed this program implemented it in 1992 in its service area that included many neighborhoods in Philadelphia with high infant mortality rates. The program was fully implemented in 1993, using strategies proven effective by home health visiting programs for high-risk infants throughout North America and abroad.

This program is designed to provide home visiting follow-up to newborns identified as high risk, either at the time of hospital discharge or at a newborn home visit during the first year of life.

■ HIGH-RISK NEWBORN FOLLOW-UP PROGRAM

Criteria for Admission

The criteria for admission to the program incorporate those risk factors associated with a high incidence of infant mortality and morbidity. Admission criteria for program inclusion are as follow:

1. The infant's birth weight is 1500 grams or less.

2. The infant is born to a mother who is 17 years old or younger.

3. The infant is born to a mother who received no prenatal care, had less than 4 prenatal visits, or began prenatal care in the third trimester.

4. The newborn or mother has a positive urine drug screen or there is maternal drug or alcohol abuse.

5. The newborn or mother is infected with HIV.

6. Acceptance into the program has been deemed medically necessary by the pediatric care provider.

Initial Newborn Home Visit

1. The first home visit will be completed within 24–72 hours of discharge as determined by medical condition at hospital discharge.

2. The following paperwork is to be completed and submitted to the office:

   a. Consent for Treatment, Release of Information, Assignment of Benefits, Notice of Client Rights. Copies of these forms should also be provided to the client.

   b. Newborn Universal Home Assessment Tool

   c. Plan of Care

   d. Clinical Time Log/Encounter Form

Cases Eligible for the High-Risk Newborn Follow-up Program

1. Newborns identified as high risk at the time of the newborn referral or newborn visit are eligible for the program.

2. A Comprehensive Initial Evaluation Visit is necessary and entails the following:

   a. A Comprehensive Evaluation Visit will be scheduled within one week of the first newborn home visit for those infants admitted to the High-Risk Newborn Home Visiting program. It is recommended that all newborns receive access to at least one visit in order to assure universal home risk assessment. Not all newborns receiving access to universal home risk assessment will be admitted to the High-Risk Newborn Home Visiting Follow-Up Program. For those newborns fitting the admission criteria, this will be the second visit. Newborns not fitting the admission criteria may be discharged or may receive a home visit plan that does not necessitate a year-long follow-up program. The nurse should complete the Initial Evaluation Form and the Home Needs Assessment Tool (found in the Appendix) as part of this visit, incorporating information from the Newborn Universal Home Assessment Tool completed at the first home visit.

b. Newborns will be seen according to an individualized Plan of Care established by the pediatric care provider for the program. The Plans of Care must be reevaluated every 62 days throughout the infant's first year of life.

c. The following paperwork is to be completed and submitted to the office.

1) Consent for Treatment, Release of Information, Assignment of Benefits, Notice of Client Rights. Copies of these forms should also be provided to the client.

2) Initial Evaluation Form

3) Home Needs Assessment Form

4) Plan of Care for first 62 days

5) Clinical Time Log/Encounter Form

3. Follow-up visits

a. Follow-up visits will be performed according to the Standard Plans of Care or any addenda ordered by the pediatric care provider.

b. The following paperwork is to be completed and submitted to the office:

1) Nursing Plan of Care and Progress Record

2) Clinical Time Log/Encounter Form

3) Revised Plan of Treatment every 62 days

4. Deviations from standard protocol
Every attempt should be made to see newborns according to the visit frequency established in the Plan of Care. If this does not occur, an addendum to the Plan of Treatment must be completed by the nurse and forwarded to the pediatric care provider for his or her signature.

5. The nurse should know the proper person to contact when a problem arises.

a. The clinical administrator should be contacted for any patient care or health status questions, or before referrals to a child protective agency.

b. The business manager should be contacted for any questions or concerns regarding the health insurance status of the client. He or she should be notified immediately of any changes in health insurance to ensure reimbursement for all nursing visits.

c. The administrative secretary should be contacted regarding any questions or changes to the client visit schedule or when a client requires assistance in accessing community resources.

d. The pediatric care provider should be notified of any abnormalities or deteriorations of health status noted at the time of the client visit. If the nurse is unsure whether or not to notify the pediatric care provider, the clinical administrator should be consulted.

Discharge Criteria

Newborns will be discharged from the program for any of the following reasons:

1. Insurance changed or denied: The newborn's insurance has changed to a payor who does not reimburse for the program or prior authorization of the services has been denied.

2. Unable to locate: After repeated attempts, the newborn cannot be located.

3. Refused visits: The caregiver has refused to continue visits for the newborn.

4. Noncompliance

5. Goals met: The newborn has reached the first birthday and achieved the goals stated in the Plan of Care.

6. Rehospitalized: The newborn has been admitted to the hospital for two weeks or longer.

7. Moved out of service area: The newborn's family has moved outside of the agency's service area.

8. Transferred: The newborn has been transferred to the care of another home health agency.

9. Placed or adopted: The newborn has been placed in foster care or adopted.

10. Expired

Data Collection

Information regarding the newborn referrals and their disposition is collected and reported on a monthly and quarterly basis. A program summary should be prepared annually and presented to the professional advisory committee. Data collection forms can be found in the Appendix.

The number of newborns admitted to the home care program should correspond to the geographic area's newborn mortality rate (that is, if the agency visits a geographic area with a newborn mortality rate of 15%, the number admitted to high-risk newborn home care identified through universal screening should reflect a similar percentage).

High-Risk Home Visiting Follow-up Plan

Box 3-1 is an actual schedule of visits and what is entailed at each visit. Visits may be done by a nurse–social worker team or by the nurse alone (in this case the nurse must have community resource experience). For this reason, some visits will mention a social worker's presence.

BOX 3-1: HOME VISIT SCHEDULE

Content of Visit	Timing of Home Visit	Key Points to Evaluate (No Complications)	Key Points to Evaluate (Special Care Infants)
The nurse should assess, observe, and evaluate the medical, psychosocial, and developmental status of the mother and newborn. Plan and provide interventions for identified problems. Assess client's educational needs and skills to perform technical care. Provide guidance in caregiver skills involving feeding, nutrition, breastfeeding support, normal and abnormal behavior development needs, and danger signs. Assist with coordination of equipment, medical supplies, prescriptions, emergency plan, and WIC screens.	24–72 hours after discharge for maternal–newborn clients without delivery/postpartum/neonatal problems. 24 hours after discharge for maternal–newborn clients with delivery/postpartum/neonatal complications.	At discharge, the nurse should perform the following tasks. 1. Identify pediatric provider. 2. Assess medical needs. 3. Intervene if there are any medical problems. 4. Determine social/support needs. 5. Identify the necessary medical equipment and supplies. 6. Schedule appointments: WIC (if eligible), pediatric provider, insurance. 7. Assist with prescription problems. 8. Identify special needs.	At discharge, the nurse should perform the following tasks. 1. Identify pediatric provider. 2. Assess medical needs. 3. Intervene if there are any medical problems. 4. Determine social/support needs. 5. Identify the necessary medical equipment and supplies. 6. Schedule appointments: WIC (if eligible), pediatric provider, insurance. 7. Assist with prescription problems. 8. Identify special needs.
The nurse or social worker should assess, observe, evaluate, and plan and provide interventions for identified problems. An individual needs-based plan should be developed.	1 week after discharge	1. The infant's appointment with the pediatric provider should be made. 2. Assess growth and development, and physical status. 3. Assist in scheduling WIC appointment, if eligible. 4. Identify appointments not made and help facilitate appointments. 5. Identify individual social problems. Facilitate resolution. 6. Assess the need for welfare, family planning, and pediatric provider. 7. Assist with access to public or low cost child health insurance, if needed.	1. The infant's appointment with the pediatric provider should be made. 2. Assess growth and development, and physical status. 3. Assist in scheduling WIC appointment, if eligible. 4. Identify appointments not made and help facilitate appointments. 5. Identify individual social problems. Facilitate resolution. 6. Assess the need for welfare, family planning, and pediatric provider. 7. Assist with access to public or low cost child health insurance, if needed. 8. Infant high risk appointment. 9. Check medical supplies and medicinal needs.

The nurse should assess, observe, and evaluate the medical, psychosocial, and developmental status. Plan and provide interventions for identified problems. Monitor health and resolution of identified problems. Provide teaching based on appropriate feeding, newborn weight gain, development, parenting, infant behaviors, maternal feelings, safety, car seats, bath safety, and hygiene.	Visits weekly between 2 and 4 weeks	1. Pediatric provider, 2 weeks. 2. Maternal WIC appointment, if eligible, 3 weeks. 3. Pediatric WIC appointment, if eligible, 3 weeks. 4. Assess growth and development.	1. Pediatric provider, 2 weeks. 2. Maternal WIC appointment, if eligible, 3 weeks. 3. Pediatric WIC appointment, if eligible, 3 weeks. 4. Assess growth and development. 5. Assess need for medical supplies, equipment, and prescriptions.
The nurse or social worker should assess, observe, evaluate, and plan and provide interventions for identified problems. Provide direct assistance with identified barriers to healthcare. Monitoring identified problems, appropriate behaviors, developments, and parental attachment. Assure access to health insurance for mother and/or infant and/or budgeting of welfare benefits.	5 weeks after discharge	1. Follow up on insurance coverage if it continues to be a problem. 2. Pediatric provider, 5 weeks. 3. Family planning, 6 weeks. 4. Assess growth and development.	1. Follow up on insurance coverage if it continues to be a problem. 2. Pediatric provider, 5 weeks. 3. Family planning, 6 weeks. 4. Assess growth and development. 5. Assess need for medical supplies, equipment, and prescriptions. 6. Determine if the infant is being followed through a high risk infant hospital program and establish communication with the neonatologist, if the infant is enrolled in this type of program.
The nurse should assess, observe, and evaluate the medical, psychosocial, and developmental status. Plan and provide interventions for identified problems. Monitor the health of the mother and infant. Reinforce and facilitate family planning; instruct about infant weight gain, immunizations, vision, and hearing. Monitor safety, safety hazards, nutrition/feeding, child/day care, the health of the family, dental, vision, hearing, and danger signs. Identify the maternal primary care provider.	8 weeks after discharge	1. Maternal primary provider appointment, 9 weeks. 2. WIC appointment, if eligible, 8 weeks. 3. Pediatric provider appointment, 8-9 weeks (immunizations). 4. Assess growth and development.	1. Maternal primary provider appointment, 9 weeks. 2. WIC appointment, if eligible, 8 weeks. 3. Pediatric provider appointment, 8-9 weeks (immunizations). 4. Assess growth and development. 5. Assess need for medical supplies, equipment, and prescriptions.

(continued)

BOX 3-1: HOME VISIT SCHEDULE (continued)

Content of Visit	Timing of Home Visit	Key Points to Evaluate (No Complications)	Key Points to Evaluate (Special Care Infants)
The nurse should assess, observe, and evaluate the medical, psychosocial, and developmental status. Plan and provide interventions for identified problems. Monitor health status and access to care. Educate parents concerning fire safety, electric, stress, feeding, nutrition, general family safety, poison, hygiene, and allergies. Assess medicinal needs and immunizations.	12–16 weeks after discharge	1. Pediatric provider appointment (immunizations), 3–4 months. 2. Assess growth and development.	1. Pediatric provider appointment (immunizations), 3-4 months. 2. Assess growth and development. 3. Assess need for medical supplies, equipment, and prescriptions.
The nurse should assess, observe, and evaluate the medical, psychosocial, and developmental status. Plan and provide interventions for identified problems. Monitor health status. Provide resources to the mother as desired: education, jobs, day care, Head Start, home safety, environmental, infant behaviors, development, parenting, stress, and immunization status.	16–20 weeks after discharge	1. Pediatric provider appointment, 5 months. 2. WIC appointment, if eligible, 5 months. 3. Assess growth and development.	1. Pediatric provider appointment, 5 months. 2. WIC appointment, if eligible, 5 months. 3. Assess growth and development.
The nurse or social worker should assess, observe, and evaluate the medical, psychosocial, and developmental status. Plan and provide interventions for identified problems. Reassess plan, and determine the need to reassess welfare. Evaluate parenting skills and budgeting.	25–26 weeks	1. Pediatric provider appointment (immunizations), 6 months. 2. WIC appointment, if eligible, 6 and 7 months. 3. Assess growth and development.	1. Pediatric provider appointment (immunizations), 6 months. 2. WIC appointment, if eligible, 6 and 7 months. 3. Return to high risk clinic. 4. Assess growth and development. 5. Assess the need for medical supplies, equipment, and prescriptions.

The nurse will focus on the provision of assessments and interventions which will identify problems requiring early intervention. Evaluate the effectiveness of the nursing service provided each visit. Focus with the family on education, centered on the emotional and developmental needs of the family/infant.	29–30 weeks	1. Pediatric provider appointment (immunizations), 8 months. 2. WIC appointment, if eligible, 8 months. 3. Assess growth and development.	1. Pediatric provider appointment (immunizations), 8 months. 2. WIC appointment, if eligible, 8 months. 3. Assess growth and development. 4. Assess the need for medical supplies, equipment, and prescriptions.
The nurse will assess, observe, and evaluate the medical, psychosocial, and developmental status. Plan and provide interventions for identified problems. Monitor health, hearing, vision, feeding, nutrition, appropriate behaviors, and development. Assess the need for primary care of other family members and public health issues.	35–37 weeks	1. Pediatric provider appointment (immunizations), 10 months. 2. WIC appointments, if eligible, 7–12 months. 3. Assess growth and development.	1. Pediatric provider appointment (immunizations), 10 months. 2. WIC appointments, if eligible, 7–12 months. 3. Assess growth and development. 4. Assess the need for medical supplies, equipment, and prescriptions.
The nurse will assess, observe, and evaluate the medical, psychosocial, and developmental status. Plan and provide interventions for identified problems. Monitor health status of infant/family. Teach home safety, cleaning items, food storage, safety locks, steps, and swimming pools. Reenforce both electric and fire safety. Teach appropriate behaviors for age.	41–43 weeks.	1. Pediatric provider appointment (immunizations), 11 months. 2. WIC appointment, if eligible.	1. Pediatric provider appointment (immunizations), 11 months. 2. WIC appointment, if eligible. 3. Assess growth and development. 4. Assess the need for medical supplies, equipment, and prescriptions.
The nurse will assess, observe, and evaluate the medical, psychosocial, and developmental status. Plan and provide interventions for identified problems. Monitor health status/follow-up of problems, age-appropriate behavior, stress, nutrition, feeding, safety (cribs, furniture, outlets) and follow-up health care plans designed for family. Reinforce healthy environments, immunizations, and discharge to the care of a physician.	43–52 weeks.	1. Pediatric provider appointment (immunizations), 12 months. 2. WIC appointment, if eligible. 3. Assess growth and development.	1. Pediatric provider appointment (immunizations), 12 months. 2. WIC appointment, if eligible. 3. Assess growth and development. 4. Assess the need for medical supplies, equipment, and prescriptions. 5. Return to high risk clinic, if enrolled.

■ HIGH-RISK FOLLOW-UP OUTCOME MEASURES

GOAL	MEASUREMENT

BIRTH to 2 MONTHS

GOAL	MEASUREMENT
Linkage to health care system and PCP (pediatric care provider) identified	Family knows health care provider's name, phone number, and how to make appointment
Newborn home visits	Appointment kept
Initial newborn visit (PCP)	At least 1 newborn visit appointment kept
ER use and rehospitalization minimized	No inappropriate ER visits or preventable hospitalizations

Social/Financial Support

GOAL	MEASUREMENT
Health insurance for newborn	Child has health insurance, private or through state
Adequate maternal food	Has access to balanced diet and food stamps
Adequate infant food	Has access to breastfeeding or formula
WIC referral and appointment (if eligible)	WIC appointment kept
Adequate newborn supplies	Has clothing, diapers, bottles and a place for newborn to sleep
Transportation for health care appointments	Identified source of transportation (e.g., car, bus, cab)
Mental health/drug/alcohol counseling	Appointment scheduled and kept
Parenting problems identified and addressed	Teaching initiated; referrals initiated

Newborn Nutrition

GOAL	MEASUREMENT
Adequate food	Access to formula; enrolled in WIC
Appropriate weight gain	Weight gain of 4–6 oz per week for full-term newborn and 3–4 oz per week for premature newborn
Other: list specific need	Referral or other problem solving initiated

2–4 MONTHS

Newborn Nutrition

GOAL	MEASUREMENT
Appropriate growth and weight gain	Growth consistent with weight graph
Developmental milestones reached	Documented in home care chart
Appropriate utilization of health care system	Caregiver is compliant with appointments
Appointment for immunizations kept	Immunizations received on schedule
Lead level determined	Lead level known
Enrolled in EPSDT program (if eligible)	Receiving care from EPSDT provider

Social/Financial Support

GOAL	MEASUREMENT
Referrals previously initiated in place	Appointments kept
Other: list specific need	
Referral or other problem solving initiated	

(continued)

GOAL	**MEASUREMENT**

4–6 MONTHS

Newborn Nutrition

Appropriate growth and weight gain	Growth consistent with weight graph
Nutritional support and teaching	Documented in home care chart
Transition from formula to baby food begun	Documented in home care chart
Developmental milestones reached	Documented in home care chart
Appropriate utilization of health care system	Caregiver is compliant with appointments
Appointment for immunizations kept	Immunizations received on schedule
Lead level drawn at 6 mos	Lead level known

Social/Financial Support

Referrals previously initiated in place	Appointments kept
Other: List specific need	Referral or other problem solving initiated

6–8 MONTHS

Newborn Nutrition

Appropriate growth and weight gain	Growth consistent with weight graph
Developmental milestones reached	Documented in home care chart

Social/Financial Support

Any outstanding problems addressed	Documented in home care chart
Other: list specific need	Referral or other problem solving initiated

8–10 MONTHS

Newborn Nutrition

Appropriate growth and weight gain	Growth consistent with weight graph
Developmental milestones reached	Documented in home care chart
Appropriate utilization of health care system	Caregiver is compliant with appointments
Lead level drawn by 9 mos	If first lead level known, result was $>$10–14 μg/dl

Social/Financial Support

Any outstanding problems addressed	Documented in home care chart
Other: list specific need	Referral or other problem solving initiated

10–12 MONTHS

Newborn Nutrition

Appropriate growth and weight gain	Growth consistent with weight graph
Developmental milestones reached	Documented in home care chart
Appropriate utilization of health care system	Caregiver is compliant with appointments
Adequately immunized	All first year immunizations received
Lead level drawn by 12 mos	If first lead level known, result was $>$10 μg/dl

Social/Financial Support

Any outstanding problems addressed	Documented in home care chart
Other: list specific need	Referral or other problem solving initiated
Discharge planning	Any ongoing needs and sources of support are documented in the home care chart

CHAPTER 4

Invasive Procedures

As part of a comprehensive home care program for the high-risk newborn, it is frequently necessary for the nurse to perform invasive procedures. These procedures can be as routine as obtaining a follow-up metabolic screening specimen required by the pediatric care provider and the state in which the baby is born. Home care providers should familiarize themselves with the laws of their individual state.

Another invasive procedure that is frequently performed in the newborn is the collection of blood specimens for the evaluation of bilirubin levels. Bilirubin, a waste product given off by the expired red blood cell, whose life expectancy is only about 2 days, is eliminated from the system through the liver. A newborn liver takes several days to mature to the point of being able to perform this function. As a result, bilirubin levels continue to increase each day of life after birth until the liver begins to eliminate it from the body.

On rare occasions the bilirubin levels will exceed accepted normals, placing the newborn at severe neurologic risk. In order to prevent this problem, bilirubin specimens are usually drawn on any babies showing signs of jaundice from hyperbilirubinemia prior to hospital discharge. However, since jaundice is frequently not seen until after discharge from the hospital (due to the etiology), the home care nurse may be the first to note it and may obtain a specimen in the home. Therefore home care nurses must be prepared to obtain the appropriate specimen if indicated.

Bilirubin levels must be followed over several days until values begin to drop back to normal levels indicating increasing liver function, or until levels continue to rise to the point that home phototherapy must be instituted. Nursing protocols specific to home phototherapy services are included in a later chapter of this manual.

Other newborns might require home intravenous therapy. In most instances, this would be preventive therapy, but it could also serve to complete a 7- to 10-day course of antibiotics initiated in the hospital.

Nurses must have adequate training and experience before performing any of these invasive procedures in the home independently. Strict aseptic technique must be practiced in order to prevent infection.

COLLECTION AND RECORDING OF BLOOD SPECIMENS FOR METABOLIC SCREENING

POLICY: A blood specimen for metabolic screening will be obtained from the infant's heel.

PURPOSE: The specimen will be obtained to fulfill state requirements for metabolic screening tests.

PROCEDURE:

1. The agency will verify the need for a metabolic screen with the pediatric care provider for babies discharged 24 hours after birth.

2. The nurse assigned to visit the infant will be responsible for filling in the following information on the screening form.

   a. Name

   b. Address

   c. Date and time of birth

   d. Facility of birth

   e. Physician

   f. Insurance company

   g. Sex, race, birth weight (in grams)

   h. Specimen purpose code

   i. County of residence

   j. Specimen date and time

3. The metabolic specimen is to be collected using the procedure for heel stick. All four circles on both sides of paper are to be completely filled with blood. (When done correctly, blood will seep through front to back.)

4. On the clinical record, document the metabolic screen done and the name of the health care provider giving the order.

5. The specimen must dry thoroughly in the dark for 4 hours before being placed in a wax envelope. (For drying in the dark, a shoe box is suggested.)

6. All completed specimens are to be mailed to the agency on the same day as drawn, or as soon as the specimen has dried adequately.

7. The agency will send copies of the physician's portion of the form to the physician when secured from the laboratory.

8. If a repeat screening is necessary, the pediatric care provider must be contacted for the order and repeat test must be recorded in the metabolic screening book alongside the original. The repeat metabolic screening lab number and date must be recorded.

9. The agency will send the specimen to the state laboratory.

10. The results will be posted in the metabolic screening tracking log.

11. Abnormal levels will be immediately reported to the pediatric care provider.

BLOOD SAMPLE COLLECTION BY HEEL OR FINGER STICK

POLICY:

- A blood sample will be drawn per order.

- Lab results must be noted and reported to the pediatric health care provider to determine if follow-up treatment is necessary.

PURPOSE:

Blood will be drawn obtain an acceptable serum sample to be transported to the laboratory for testing.

EQUIPMENT NEEDED:

1. Alcohol swabs

2. Foot/finger warmer (a warm wash cloth or disposable diaper may also be used.)

3. Sterile lancet

4. Appropriate collection tube (check with the lab performing the test)

5. Band-aid

6. 2 × 2 gauze square

7. Vaseline (optional)

8. Labels

9. Clean gloves

PROCEDURE:

1. You must first receive a referral from the office.

2. Contact the parents by phone to arrange the time of the visit.

3. Explain to the parents that you are going to take a small amount of blood from their child and that they may leave the room if they wish.

4. Expose the infant's foot.

5. Wrap the heel in the foot warmer and allow adequate time for the heel to warm (3 to 5 minutes).

6. Place the infant on a flat surface where he or she will be safe from falling.

7. Put on clean gloves.

8. Remove the warmer and select the puncture site. Cleanse with the site with an alcohol swab. (Optional: Dab on a thin layer of Vaseline.)

9. Puncture the skin with a sterile lancet.

10. Wipe away the first drop of blood with a sterile 2×2 gauze pad.

11. If using a microtainer, follow these steps:
    a. Hold the microtainer tube with the Flo Top collector at an angle below horizontal with the vent hole in an upward position.
    b. Touch the tip of the Flo Top collector to the underside of the drop of blood. Blood will flow freely through the Flo Top collector.
    c. Upon termination of the collecting procedure, wipe the wound dry and cover with a Band-aid.
    d. Twist off the Flo Top collector from the tube and discard.
    e. Put a plug securely in the tube opening and label the tube with the infant's name.

12. Inform the parents that you are going to transport the blood sample to the hospital, that the home care agency office will call them with the results, and that their pediatric care provider will also be notified.

13. Call the office with your report of the assessment and the lab drop-off time.

14. Take the blood sample directly to the lab. Protect specimens from sunlight by placing them in a thick padded envelope.

15. Provide the lab with the necessary patient information and request that they call the home care agency office as well as the pediatric care provider's office with the results.

RECOMMENDATIONS FOR SKIN PUNCTURES IN NEWBORNS:

1. Perform heel punctures on the most medial or most lateral portion of the plantar surface of the foot.

2. Puncture no deeper than 2.4 mm.

3. Do not perform punctures on the posterior curvature of the heel.

4. Do not puncture through previous sites that may be infected.

5. For finger stick, use most lateral portions of the palmar side of the third or fourth fingertips.

POLICY AND PROCEDURE: PERIPHERAL VENIPUNCTURE TO INSERT A CATHETER

POLICY: The nurse will maintain the patency of the peripheral line for infusion therapy, as prescribed.

PURPOSE: Maintenance of peripheral patency will permit the prescribed administration of fluids and medication on a continuous or intermittent basis.

EQUIPMENT NEEDED:

1. Tape (clear tape on babies under 3 years old). Nonallergic tape should be used with excoriated skin.

2. Intravenous cannula as appropriate

3. Sharps container

4. Normal saline

5. Latex gloves

6. Heparinized saline concentration

7. Transparent dressing

8. Injection cap

9. Alcohol swabs

10. Povidone–iodine swabs

FREQUENCY: Intravenous site rotation should occur every 3 days, or more often as needed for phlebitis, thrombosis, infiltration, infection, or other problems (unless otherwise ordered by health care provider).

PROCEDURE:

1. Explain the procedure to the parent or caregiver.

2. Prepare a clean work surface.

3. Organize the supplies needed.

4. Wash your hands (following handwashing procedure) and put on latex gloves.

5. Select IV cannulas.
   a. Butterflies
      1) 23- and 21-gauge butterflies are most frequently used.
      2) For difficult venous access, a 27- or 25-gauge butterfly may be used.

   b. Catheters

      1) Sizes range from 14- to 24-gauge catheters. The gauge of the needle depends on the newborn's needs.

      2) Catheters are used over butterflies in the following instances:

         (a) When infusing a drug or solution that is very irritating to the vein.

         (b) For infusion via pump.

6. Select insertion site.

   a. Examine all extremities for venous access.

   b. Begin examining distally and work proximally to the newborn.

   c. Only superficial veins are to be used. Veins in the leg and above the ankle are prominent in premature newborns and should not be used due to circulatory compromise of the foot.

   d. Contraindications of placement are listed below.

      1) Infection, osteomyelitis, and cellulitis—do not use affected extremity.

      2) Vasospasm secondary to deep lines with discoloration of an extremity—do not use the affected extremity.

   e. Prepare the site.

      1) Using a circular motion, cleanse first with alcohol wipes, then with a povidone–iodine swab.

      2) Allow to dry for 20 seconds.

   f. Insert cannula.

      1) Apply a tourniquet to dilate the vein.

      2) Put on latex gloves.

      3) The site may be numbed with 0.1 or 0.2 ml of normal saline intradermally, using a 27- or 26-gauge needle (optional).

      4) Hold the catheter comfortably and firmly for insertion and secure the vein below the insertion site with the other hand.

      5) Insert the needle, bevel up, through the skin parallel to the vein, until blood return is achieved. Thread cannula until the hub is proximal to the skin surface. **Note:** Pre-sticking with a 21- or 22-gauge needle for a 22- or 24-gauge catheter may be done to ease insertion (optional).

      6) No more than three attempts may be made by one nurse. Table 4-1 shows some common problems that can arise and solutions for these problems.

      7) Secure the cannula in place with tape.

         (a) Do not apply tape too tightly because pressure sores may occur, especially under the hub of the catheter.

         (b) Do not place tape directly over the site.

         (c) Apply povidone–iodine ointment to all catheters and a transparent dressing over the insertion site.

      8) Remove the tourniquet and stylet.

9) Connect either intravenous tubing or an injection cap (heparin lock) into the cannula and secure.

    (a) For an injection cap (heparin lock), flush with heparin and check for patency by aspirating for blood return and observe for signs/symptoms of infiltration.

    (b) In giving a medication dose, the heparin lock is flushed with 0.3 ml of normal saline. Administer the medication, then 0.3 ml of normal saline flush after the medication dose, then the heparin flush (1 ml normal saline/10 units of heparin solution).

    (c) Minimum flushing of injection cap (heparin lock) is once per day when not in use.

10) Document the insertion site, gauge of catheter, date and time of insertion, nurse's initials, and any complications of the procedure. This should be noted on the nursing progress notes.

11) Inform the patient and parent or caregiver of signs and symptoms of complications and rationale and performance of this procedure as appropriate.

12) Discard all used materials in sharps container.

TABLE 4-1
Guidelines for Problematic Patient Conditions

Patient Condition	Effect on Patient	Guidelines
Shock; sepsis, hypotension	Poor perfusion, vasoconstriction, difficult to locate veins	1. Flush fluid through needle 2. Use different tourniquet tensions or blood pressure cuff techniques 3. Expect no blood return 4. Inserter rarely feels needle enter the vein 5. Soaks may help but are not very effective 6. Squeeze distally and proximally to site at the same time to pump up the vein
Increased temp., febrile	Dilated veins	1. May not get blood return 2. Usually easier to find veins
Decreased body temperature due to: cold environment, use of cooling mattress, use of multiple swabs with alcohol on babies	Vasoconstriction	1. Apply warm soaks over a large area 2. Wrap with blanket and wait 30 minutes 3. Use warmer bed if available 4. Use different tourniquet tensions or blood pressure cuff techniques 5. Expect minimal blood return
Fear vasoconstriction	Fight or flight	1. Control breathing; insert needle when patient is exhaling 2. Have patient blow out candles or shout Ouch!
Jaundice or bililights (phototherapy), low platelets	Fragile veins	1. Apply low tourniquet tension 2. Insert needle into vein slowly and advance gently 3. Remove tourniquet rapidly
Malnutrition: poor skin turgor, poor muscle tone	Large, unstabilized veins	1. Exaggerate skin tension 2. Insert whole unit in the vein before advancing the catheter
Flaccidity: very poor muscle tone, loose skin	Rolling veins not visible or palpable	1. Rely on anatomy 2. Exaggerate skin tension 3. Using the veins of the feet is usually easier
Obesity	Veins not visible	1. Digital veins are often visible 2. Rely on anatomy
Edema	Veins not visible	1. Press out fluid 2. Test for refill 3. Insert needle far enough into the vein so that returning fluid will not push the needle out
Long-term therapy	Damaged veins; many collateral veins	1. Use any necessary guidelines

POLICY AND PROCEDURE: PERIPHERAL LINE AND HEPARIN LOCK APPLICATION

POLICY: The nurse will insert and maintain heparin lock patency as prescribed.

PURPOSE: The nurse will maintain an intravenous line via a heparin lock for patients requiring venous access for medication. Allow the patient freedom of mobility.

PROCEDURE:

1. Follow nursing procedure for peripheral venipuncture, assessment of site, insertion of catheter, and taping of site.

2. Flush heparin lock with 0.5 to 1 ml of heparin flush solution (1 ml normal saline/10 units heparin solution) at the time of insertion of the heparin lock and after each dose of medication.

3. In giving the medication dose, the heparin lock is flushed with 0.3 ml of normal saline. Administer the medication, then 0.3 ml of normal saline flush after the medication dose, then the heparin flush (1 ml normal saline/10 units of heparin solution).

4. Assess the intravenous site at the time of flushing for infiltration, phlebitis, and/or leaking.

5. Document on the Nursing Medication Sheet and Nursing Progress Notes the following information.

    a. Date and time heparin lock was started

    b. Date and time site was changed

    c. Gauge of intravenous needle

    d. Medication administered

    e. Assessment of site

6. Properly discard all materials in sharps container.

7. Educate family member or caregiver in the procedure for applying pressure to the site if the heparin lock should become dislodged.

▨ POLICY AND PROCEDURE: PERIPHERAL INTRAVENOUS COMPLICATIONS

POLICY: The nurse should be able to recognize signs and symptoms of peripheral intravenous therapy complications.

PURPOSE: Expedient recognition will allow the nurse to apply the appropriate intervention for complications of intravenous therapy.

PROCEDURE:

1. Phlebitis: Inflammation of the walls of the vein.

   a. *Cause:* Direct injury/trauma to the vein from intravenous injections, indwelling catheters, overuse of a vein, infusion of an irritating solution, use of a large-bore cannula, long-term cannula placement, or extension of an infection into the tissue surrounding the vessel.

   b. *Symptoms:* Venous distention, edema, local heat, erythema, induration, or pain at the site of cannula placement and along the course of the affected vein.

   c. *Intervention:* Identify and document the symptoms. Change the IV site. Apply cold compresses for 24 hours, with moist heat thereafter to stimulate circulation and promote absorption. Continue observation for elevated temperature, purulence, pain, erythema, or local heat at the identified site. Notify the health care provider of the intervention and obtain further prescribed orders.

2. Thrombosis: Clot formation in the cannula or vessel that occludes flow through the catheter or vessel.

   a. *Cause:* Usually caused by stasis of blood in catheter by patient position or neglectful heparinization of the catheter.

   b. *Symptoms:* Inability to flush catheter, erythema, inflammation, induration of insertion site.

   c. *Intervention:* Discontinue peripheral intravenous line according to procedure. Notify the health care provider and proceed as prescribed.

3. Infiltration: Accumulation of fluid in tissue surrounding intravenous cannula.

   a. *Cause:* Dislocation of cannula or loss of vessel integrity.

   b. *Symptoms:* Edema, skin blanching, pain, decreased temperature of skin at the site as well as slowing or cessation of intravenous fluid not associated with mechanical or tubing problems. **Note:** A blood return may still be present with infiltration.

   c. *Intervention:* Discontinue infusion and cannula. Apply warm compresses to site of infiltrate to increase fluid absorption. Notify health care provider and proceed as prescribed.

4. Embolism: Obstruction of a blood vessel by a blood clot or a foreign substance.

   a. *Cause:* Most common cause is dislodging of a thrombus into systemic circulation.

   b. *Symptoms:* Ischemia, hypotension, dyspnea, cyanosis, tachycardia, peripheral numbness, tingling, and loss of consciousness.

   c. *Intervention:* Call health care provider immediately and initiate emergency procedure, as should be stated in the policies of all providers of this service. ***Note:*** If a catheter fragment has entered the systemic circulation, immediately apply firm pressure (proximal manual tourniquet) to contain the fragment.

5. Infection: Intravenous site that has been invaded by pathogenic organisms producing deleterious effects locally and systemically.

   a. *Cause:* Poor aseptic technique, contamination of the catheter and/or solution, and intrinsic factors (immunosuppression, steroid therapy, or malnutrition)

   b. *Symptoms:* Fever, chills, tachycardia, erythema, inflammation, purulence, pain, and localized heat from insertion site

   c. *Intervention:* Prevent infection by inspecting solution and supplies for contamination. Properly review and practice aseptic techniques. Notify health care provider of signs and symptoms and proceed with prescribed orders.

TEACHING CAREGIVERS AND PATIENTS:

1. For all of the complications described above, the caregivers and patients are to be educated concerning the following information.

   a. The condition and the definition of the condition

   b. Symptomatology

   c. Proper interventions

2. All teaching by the infusion nurse should be documented and reviewed at each visit.

POLICY AND PROCEDURE: DISCONTINUATION OF PERIPHERAL INTRAVENOUS CATHETER

POLICY:
The nurse will discontinue the peripheral intravenous catheter properly when prescribed.

PURPOSE:
An intravenous cannula will be removed when intravenous access is no longer prescribed, when site rotation is necessary, or when complications exist.

PROCEDURE:

1. Place gauze over the site of the cannula insertion and withdraw cannula.

2. Hold the gauze in place with slight pressure being applied for 2 to 3 minutes.

3. Check the site for continued bleeding. ***Note:*** If bleeding continues, apply pressure or pressure dressing.

4. If there is no bleeding, apply a bandage or gauze with tape.

5. Discard all materials in sharps container.

6. Document on the Nursing Progress Notes the time, date, and assessment of the site after discontinuation.

CHAPTER 5

Specific Protocols for High-Risk Newborn Follow-Up

The following section of this manual provides specific protocols that address the most common medical maladies that can affect the high-risk newborn. These protocols were designed and used in the provision of newborn care in the home. They have been developed over the course of 7 years and have been reviewed, revised, and approved by home health agency clinical advisory staff made up of experts in the field of maternal–child health.

The protocols should be copied and used in the orientation of all nursing staff. They also provide a quick and easy guide that nurses in the field can carry with them. The Initial Newborn Home Assessment Tool should be used on the first visit to enable the nurse to provide appropriate risk assessment and determine the level of care based on those findings. Level of care determinations are categorized as level 1, 2, or 3 and help to define the number of visits necessary to attain the goals stated in the Plan of Care. The protocols should be reviewed annually by the individual home health provider's clinical advisors to assure they remain current and fulfill the requirements of federal Medicare standards, National League of Nursing criteria of certification, and the accreditation standards of the Joint Commission for Accreditation of Healthcare Organizations.

■ HOME CARE PROTOCOL: APNEA MONITOR

Eligibility Requirements

1. The initial acute treatment has been completed.

2. Laboratory test values are within the normal range.

3. A pneumogram and other pertinent sleep studies have been completed.

4. The newborn is free of infection.

5. The parents have received CPR and monitor training.

6. The newborn is receiving an adequate amount of formula to promote an average weight gain of 15 to 20 grams per 24 hours; this applies to the premature neonate only, because weight gain is not a significant indicator for discharge of the older newborn.

7. The pediatric care provider has been selected.

8. The predischarge assessment in the home has been completed.

9. All of the necessary equipment has been ordered.

10. The patient has been discharged 24 to 48 hours after meeting the discharge criteria.

11. The electric company has been notified of the medical need for power priority.

12. The appropriate utilities have been notified of the need for water, phone, electricity, and heat in cases of economic hardship.

13. An emergency transport plan is in place.

General Nursing and Pediatric Care Provider Treatment Orders

Before discharge of the patient from the hospital, a predischarge evaluation is to be completed. The Home Needs Assessment Tool found in the appendices can be used for this purpose. This evaluation entails the following:

1. Socioeconomic evaluation

2. Laboratory tests

3. Neonatal testing results (if appropriate)

4. Complete physical assessment and history to include the following information:
   a. Birth history and hospital course
   b. Appropriate identifying information
      1) Newborn's name, address, phone number
      2) Parents' names

       3) Referring pediatric care provider's name, address, phone number

       4) Insurance type and numbers

       5) Type of home care, visits, and frequency

   c. Medications and dietary/treatment orders

   d. Supplies and equipment needed

   e. Evaluation of initial visit, establishing long-term and short-term goals

   f. Signature of the pediatric nurse and date the predischarge assessment was rendered

5. The schedule of home visits by the monitor company set up to alternate with nursing visits

6. Notification of the electric company of the state of medical priority for any child using medical electrical equipment in case of a power outage

7. Notification of the appropriate utilities of the need for water, phone, electricity, and heat in cases of economic hardship

8. Establishment of an emergency transport plan with the family and the appropriate local transport team

Nursing Assessment Each Visit

The nurse will perform physical assessment and examination to evaluate the following areas:

1. Respiratory: Auscultate the lungs for rate, rhythm, and abnormal breath sounds. Observe the character of respiratory effort (retractions, grunting, or flaring).

2. Metabolic: Assess the patient's temperature and intake.

3. Gastrointestinal: Assess for vomiting, frequent loose stools, and irritation of buttocks. Weigh the newborn, measure girth, and auscultate bowel sounds.

4. Genitourinary: Determine the number of wet diapers per 24 hours.

5. Musculoskeletal: Check muscle tone, vigor of activity, and movement of all extremities.

6. Neurologic: Assess the fontanel, irritability, cry, presence of jitteriness or seizure activity.

7. Determine number of times the alarm has sounded and the reasons why.

8. Cardiovascular: Assess the heart rate, rhythm, presence of murmur, central and peripheral color, and peripheral pulses.

Activity

The child's activity should be limited to in the home and should be appropriate for the child's age and development.

Diet

1. Review the newborn's intake.

2. Formula and volume will be determined by the pediatric care provider.

Education

1. Safety
   a. Review newborn safety; identify and correct hazards in the home.
   b. Review signs of infection, feeding intolerance, and seizures with the parents.
   c. Review the monitor and CPR with the parents; assess their understanding of apnea and what happens if the alarm sounds.

2. Growth and development
   a. Review newborn development and stimulation to promote growth.
   b. Reinforce the need for immunizations and follow-up visits.

3. Drugs: Educate the family concerning the signs and symptoms of adverse reactions to the medications prescribed.

4. Miscellaneous: Inform the parents of available community resources.

■ HOME CARE PROTOCOL: PREMATURITY AGA LESS THAN 1500 GRAMS

Eligibility Requirements

1. The initial acute treatment has been completed.

2. Laboratory test values are within normal values.

3. The newborn is free of infection.

4. Parents have demonstrated the ability to provide for the nutritional needs of the child.

5. The newborn has been gaining 15 to 20 grams per 24 hours on average.

6. The parents have been instructed in CPR.

7. Pneumogram thermistor and other pertinent neonatal testing has been completed.

8. The parents have been instructed in using the apnea monitor.

9. The newborn has been tolerating formula and gaining weight on full feeds (oral or nasogastric) for several days.

10. The pediatric care provider has been selected for follow-up.

11. A predischarge assessment in the home has been completed.

12. The necessary equipment has been ordered.

13. The pediatric support team has been established.

14. The necessary discharge medications have been obtained.

15. The electric company has been notified of the medical need for power priority.

16. The appropriate utilities have been notified of the need for water, phone, electricity, and heat in cases of economic hardship.

17. An emergency transport plan is in place.

18. The patient has been discharged 24 to 48 hours after meeting the discharge criteria.

General Nursing and Pediatric Care Provider Treatment Orders

Before discharge of the patient from the hospital, a predischarge evaluation is to be completed. This evaluation entails the following:

1. Socioeconomic evaluation

2. Laboratory tests

3. Neonatal testing results

4. Complete physical assessment and history to include the following information:

    a. Birth history and hospital course

    b. Appropriate identifying information

        1) Newborn's name, address, phone number

        2) Parents' names

        3) Referring pediatric care provider's name, address, phone number

        4) Insurance type and numbers

        5) Type of home care, visits, and frequency

    c. Medications and dietary/treatment orders

    d. Supplies and equipment needed

    e. Evaluation of initial visit, establishing long-term and short-term goals

    f. Signature of the pediatric nurse and date the predischarge assessment was rendered

5. Notification of the electric company of the state of medical priority for any child using medical electrical equipment in case of a power outage

6. Notification of the appropriate utilities of the need for water, phone, electricity, and heat in cases of economic hardship

7. Establishment of an emergency transport plan with the family and the appropriate local transport team

Nursing Assessment Each Visit

The nurse will perform physical assessment and examination to evaluate the following areas:

1. Cardiovascular: Assess heart rate, rhythm, and presence of murmur. Palpate peripheral pulses and observe for edema.

2. Respiratory: Auscultate breath sounds for signs of bronchospasm. Note the rate and rhythm of respirations and the character of respiratory effort. Note the color of oral mucosa and nail beds.

3. Metabolic: Assess the newborn's temperature and intake.

4. Gastrointestinal: Assess for vomiting, frequent loose stools, and irritation of the buttocks. Weigh the newborn and monitor intake.

5. Genitourinary: Determine the number of wet diapers per 24 hours.

6. Musculoskeletal: Check the muscle tone, vigor of activity, and movement of all extremities.

7. Neurologic: Assess the fontanel, irritability, cry, moro reflex, presence of jitterness or seizure activity.

8. Infectious disease: Note the presence of upper respiratory infection.

9. Psychological: Encourage and support the parents. Assess the need for respite care.

10. Measure the newborn's length and head circumference each week and plot them on the growth chart.

11. Check the newborn's weight each visit and plot it on the growth chart.

Activity

1. The newborn should engage in activity and bonding appropriate to age and development.

2. Avoid overstimulation that would lead to increased oxygen consumption.

3. Provide adequate rest periods.

4. Avoid prolonged exposure to outside during extreme cold snaps, excessive heat and humidity, and inclement weather.

5. Assess the need for the parents to enroll the newborn in an early intervention program and assist if indicated.

Diet

1. The formula amount and type will be determined by the newborn's age and size.

2. Solid foods will be introduced under the supervision of the pediatric care provider; allergy or sensitivity should be observed and noted.

Education

1. Safety: Review newborn safety; identify and correct hazards in the home.

2. Respiratory
    a. Reinforce the need to avoid contact between the child and those with infectious disease.
    b. Review the signs of illness and feeding intolerance (the pediatric care provider should be notified of these signs).
    c. Review the signs of respiratory distress and when to notify pediatric care provider.

3. Growth and development
    a. Review newborn development and stimulation to promote growth.
    b. Reinforce the need for immunizations and follow-up visits.
    c. Review the appropriate exercises.

4. Medications: Educate the family concerning the signs and symptoms of adverse reactions to medications prescribed.

5. Equipment: Review the use of the apnea monitor; reinforce CPR.

6. Family support
    a. Inform the family of available community support and assist them in referrals.
    b. Determine the need for respite care in the home by RN or LPN.

■ HOME CARE PROTOCOL: PREMATURITY AGA GREATER THAN 1500 GRAMS

Eligibility Requirements

1. The initial acute treatment has been completed.

2. Laboratory test values are within the normal range.

3. The newborn is free of infection.

4. The newborn has advanced to a weight gain of 15 to 20 grams per 24 hours on average.

5. The newborn has been tolerating formula and gaining weight, on full feeds (oral or naso-gastric) for several days.

6. Pneumogram thermistor has been completed and read by the pediatric care provider.

7. The parents have been instructed in CPR.

8. The need for the home oxygen program has been assessed.

9. The parents have completed monitor training as appropriate.

10. The pediatric care provider has been selected for follow-up.

11. All of the necessary equipment has been ordered.

12. A predischarge assessment in the home has been completed.

13. All of the necessary discharge medications have been obtained.

14. The electric company has been notified of the medical need for power priority.

15. The appropriate utilities have been notified of the need for water, phone, electricity, and heat in cases of economic hardship.

16. An emergency transport plan is in place.

17. The patient has been discharged 24 to 48 hours after meeting the discharge criteria.

General Nursing and Pediatric Care Provider Treatment Orders

Before discharge of the patient from the hospital, a predischarge evaluation is to be completed. This evaluation entails the following:

1. Socioeconomic evaluation

2. Laboratory tests

3. Neonatal testing results

4. Complete physical assessment and history to include the following:

    a. Birth history and hospital course

    b. Appropriate identifying information

        1) Newborn's name, address, phone number

        2) Parents' names

        3) Referring pediatric care provider's name, address, phone number

        4) Insurance type and numbers

        5) Type of home care, visits, and frequency

    c. Medications and dietary/treatment orders

    d. Supplies and equipment needed

    e. Evaluation of initial visit, establishing long-term and short-term goals

    f. Signature of the pediatric nurse and date the predischarge assessment was rendered

5. Notification of the electric company of the state of medical priority for any newborn using medical electrical equipment in case of a power outage

6. Notification of the appropriate utilities of the need for water, phone, electricity, and heat in cases of economic hardship

7. Establishment of an emergency transport plan with the family and the appropriate local transport team.

Nursing Assessment Each Visit

The nurse will perform physical assessment and examination to evaluate the following:

1. Cardiovascular: Assess heart rate, rhythm, and presence of murmur. Palpate peripheral pulses and observe for edema.

2. Respiratory: Auscultate breath sounds; observe rate and rhythm and character of respiratory effort. Observe oral mucosa and nail beds for color. Note the appropriate use of oxygen.

3. Metabolic: Assess the newborn's temperature and intake.

4. Gastrointestinal: Assess for vomiting, frequent loose stools, and irritation of buttocks. Weigh the infant, measure girth, and auscultate bowel sounds.

5. Genitourinary: Determine the number of wet diapers per 24 hours.

6. Musculoskeletal: Check muscle tone, vigor and activity, and movement of all extremities.

7. Neurologic: Assess the fontanel, irritability, and cry.

8. Measure length and head circumference each week and plot on the growth chart.

9. Check weight each visit and document on growth chart.

Activity

1. Feed the newborn in a comfortable position in an unrushed environment.

2. Observe the newborn during feeding for dyspnea and color changes.

3. Provide activity appropriate to age and development, with adequate rest periods.

Diet

1. Formula type and volume will be determined by the pediatric care provider.

2. Review feeding problems encountered by the parents.

Education

1. Safety
   a. Review infant safety; identify and correct hazards in the home.
   b. Review the signs of infection and feeding intolerance with the parents.

2. Respiratory
   a. Review the signs of respiratory distress with the parents and actions to be taken.
   b. Reinforce the need to avoid contact between the newborn and infectious persons.
   c. Review feeding patterns that decrease respiratory distress such as frequent burping and larger-hole nipple.

3. Growth and development
   a. Review infant development and stimulation to promote growth.
   b. Reinforce the need for immunizations and follow-up visits.
   c. Assess the need for occupational and physical therapies.

4. Medications
   a. Educate the family concerning the signs and symptoms of adverse reactions to medications prescribed.
   b. Reinforce the need to give medication on time and as ordered.

5. Supportive care
   a. Inform the parents of community resources available.
   b. Assess the need for financial assistance and make referrals.
   c. Determine the need for respite care to be provided by RN or LPN.
   d. Offer encouragement and support.

■ HOME CARE PROTOCOL: ORO-NASO-GASTRIC FEEDING

Eligibility Requirements

1. The initial acute treatment has been completed.

2. Laboratory test values are within the normal range.

3. The newborn is free of infection.

4. The parents have received instruction and can demonstrate the ability to pass the naso-gastric/oro-gastric tube safely.

5. The pediatric care provider has determined whether the newborn receives oro- or naso-gastric feeding.

6. The newborn is gaining weight, averaging 15 to 20 grams per 24 hours for 1 week before discharge, and has advanced to and tolerated full feedings for several days.

7. The discharge diet plan has been prepared.

8. A pediatric care provider has been selected for follow-up care.

9. A predischarge assessment in the home has been completed.

10. Feeding supplies have been ordered.

11. The newborn has been discharged 24 to 48 hours after meeting the discharge criteria.

12. The electric company has been notified of the medical need for power priority.

13. The appropriate utilities have been notified of the need for water, phone, electricity, and heat in cases of economic hardship.

14. An emergency transport plan is in place.

General Nursing and Pediatric Care Provider Treatment Orders

Before discharge of the newborn from the hospital, a predischarge evaluation is to be completed. This evaluation entails the following:

1. Socioeconomic evaluation

2. Laboratory tests

3. Neonatal testing results, including pneumograms where appropriate

4. Complete physical assessment and history to include the following:

    a. Pertinent past and current findings, including birth history and hospital course

    b. Appropriate identifying information

       1) Newborn's name, address, phone number

       2) Parents' names

       3) Referring pediatric care provider's name, address, phone number

       4) Insurance type and numbers

       5) Type of home care, visits, and frequency

    c. Medications, dietary plans, and activity

    d. Supplies and equipment needed

    e. Evaluation of initial visit, establishing long-term and short-term goals

    f. Signature of the pediatric nurse and date the predischarge assessment was rendered

5. Notification of the electric company of medical priority for any newborn using medical electrical equipment in case of a power outage

6. Notification of the appropriate utilities of the need for water, phone, electricity, and heat in cases of economic hardship

7. Establishment of an emergency transport plan with the family and the appropriate local transport team

Nursing Assessment Each Visit

1. The nurse will perform physical assessment and examination to evaluate the following:

    a. Cardiovascular: Auscultate heart rate and rhythm, assess for murmur, palpate peripheral pulses, and observe for edema.

    b. Respiratory: Auscultate breath sounds, note abnormal breath sounds; observe for rate, rhythm, and character of respirations; observe oral mucosa and nail beds for color. Note the appropriate use of oxygen.

    c. Metabolic: Assess the newborn's temperature and test urine for glucose and protein.

    d. Gastrointestinal: Assess for vomiting, reflux, diarrhea, and constipation. Measure girth and auscultate bowel sounds; check the infant's weight and review intake with the parents.

    e. Genitourinary: Check the number of wet diapers; observe for fluid retention.

    f. Musculoskeletal: Observe for muscle tone, activity, and equal movement of all extremities. Note any abnormal markings on body.

    g. Neurologic: Palpate fontanel. Assess hyper- or hypotonicity of extremities. Note the quality of cry and sucking ability. Assess irritability, jitteriness, or seizure activity.

    h. Measure length and head circumference each week and plot them on the growth chart.

    i. Check weight each visit and plot it on the growth chart.

2. Assess parent–newborn attachment and interaction, identifying potential or existing problems.

Activity

1. During feeding and for at least 1 hour after, place the newborn in one of the following positions:

   a. Prone position at 30° angle

   b. On the right side, lying at 30° angle

   c. Upright in infant seat or in a parent's arms

2. At nonfeeding time, activity is unrestricted.

Diet

The formula type and volume will be prescribed by the pediatric care provider.

Education

1. Feedings

   a. Review insertion of the naso-gastric or oro-gastric tube as ordered by the pediatric care provider and check for correct placement.

   b. Review the position of the newborn during and after feeding.

   c. Reinforce the need for nonnutritive sucking.

   d. Increase volume as recommended by the pediatric care provider and determined by growth.

   e. Review the signs of feeding intolerance.

   f. Remove the oro-gastric tube if the newborn is able to work it out with the tongue.

2. Safety: Review infant safety; identify and correct hazards in the home.

3. Growth and development: Review activities appropriate for infant stimulation and normal growth and development.

■ HOME CARE PROTOCOL: DRUG WITHDRAWAL/NEONATAL ABSTINENCE SYNDROME (NAS)

Eligibility Requirements

1. The initial acute treatment has been completed.

2. Laboratory test values are within the normal range.

3. The newborn is free of infection.

4. The parents are able to perform the following tasks:
   a. Care for the infant's physical and nutritional needs
   b. Administer medication correctly

5. A social service evaluation has been completed.

6. The infant is taking adequate nutrition for his or her size and averaging a weight gain of 15 to 20 grams per 24 hours over 1 week.

7. A predischarge assessment of the home has been completed.

8. The newborn has been discharged 24 to 48 hours after meeting the discharge criteria.

9. The electric company has been notified of the medical need for power priority.

General Nursing and Pediatric Care Provider Treatment Orders

Before discharge of the newborn from the hospital, a predischarge evaluation will be completed. This evaluation includes the following:

1. Socioeconomic evaluation, with definite reference to the mother's reliability and supports

2. Home health aide needs based upon assessment of the mother's reliability and supports

3. Laboratory test results

4. Neonatal testing results

5. Complete physical assessment and history to include the following areas:
   a. Birth history and hospital course
   b. Appropriate identifying information
      1) Newborn's name, address, phone number
      2) Parents' names
      3) Referring pediatric care provider's name, address, phone number
      4) Insurance type and numbers
      5) Type of home care, visits, and frequency

c. Medications and dietary/treatment orders

d. Supplies and equipment needed

e. Evaluation of initial visit, establishing long-term and short-term goals

f. Signature of the pediatric nurse and date the predischarge assessment was rendered

6. Notification of the electric company of the state of medical priority for any newborn using medical electrical equipment in case of a power outage

7. Notification of the appropriate utilities of the need for water, phone, electricity, and heat in cases of economic hardship

8. Establishment of an emergency transport plan with the family and the appropriate local transport team.

Nursing Assessment Each Visit

The nurse will perform physical assessment and examination to evaluate the following:

1. Cardiovascular: Assess heart rate, rhythm, and presence of murmur. Palpate peripheral pulses and observe for edema. Note the skin color for any molting.

2. Respiratory: Auscultate lungs for rate, rhythm, and abnormal breath sounds. Observe the character of respiratory effort (retractions, grunting, or flaring).

3. Metabolic: Assess the newborn's temperature and intake.

4. Gastrointestinal: Assess for vomiting, frequent loose stools, and irritation of buttocks. Weigh the infant, measure girth, and auscultate bowel sounds. Note that constipation may indicate overuse of paregoric.

5. Genitourinary: Determine the number of wet diapers per 24 hours.

6. Musculoskeletal: Check muscle tone, vigor of activity, and movement of all extremities.

7. Neurologic: Assess the fontanel, irritability, cry, moro reflex, presence of jitters, or seizure activity, inability to quiet, yawning, or sneezing.

Activity

1. Stimulation by excess noise and activity should be minimized.

2. The infant should be kept swaddled in a quiet room with subdued lights.

3. Review measures for minimizing irritability.

Diet

1. Daily quantity will be determined by the pediatric care provider.

2. Document the formula amount and number of feeds per day.

3. Burp frequently to minimize vomiting.

Education

1. Safety

    a. Review infant safety; identify and correct hazards in the home.

    b. Review the signs of infection, feeding intolerance, and seizures with parents.

2. Growth and development

    a. Review infant development and stimulation to promote growth.

    b. Reinforce the need for immunizations and follow-up visits.

3. Drugs: Educate the family concerning the signs and symptoms of adverse reactions to any medication prescribed.

4. Social: Follow up and provide a social service evaluation if there is a drug dependence situation in the family.

5. Miscellaneous: Inform the parents of the community resources available.

■ HOME CARE PROTOCOL: FAILURE TO THRIVE (NONORGANIC)

Eligibility Requirements

1. The initial acute treatment has been completed and a determination of etiology has been made.

2. Laboratory test values are within the normal range.

3. The newborn is free of infection.

4. The newborn has demonstrated an adequate weight gain with the appropriate caloric intake over several days.

5. The parents have demonstrated the ability to perform the following tasks:

    a. Feed the newborn and care for other physical needs (warmth, dryness, cleanliness)

    b. Interact with the newborn in a nurturing manner

6. A pediatric care provider has been selected.

7. A predischarge assessment in the home has been completed.

8. The electric company has been notified of the medical need for power priority.

9. The appropriate utilities have been notified of the need for water, phone, electricity, and heat in cases of economic hardship.

10. An emergency transport plan is in place.

11. The patient has been discharged 24 to 48 hours after meeting the discharge criteria.

General Nursing and Pediatric Care Provider Treatment Orders

Before discharge of the infant from the hospital, a predischarge evaluation is to be completed. The Home Needs Assessment Tool in the Appendices may be used for this purpose. This evaluation entails the following:

1. Socioeconomic evaluation

2. Laboratory tests

3. Complete physical assessment and history to include the following information:

    a. Birth history and hospital course

    b. Appropriate identifying information

        1) Newborn's name, address, phone number

        2) Parents' names

        3) Referring pediatric care provider's name, address, phone number

          4) Insurance type and numbers

          5) Type of home care, visits, and frequency

    c. Medications and dietary/treatment orders

    d. Supplies and equipment needed

    e. Evaluation of initial visit, establishing long-term and short-term goals

    f. Signature of the pediatric nurse and date the predischarge assessment was rendered

4. Notification of the electric company of medical priority for any newborn using medical electrical equipment in case of a power outage

5. Notification of the appropriate utilities of the need for water, phone, electricity, and heat in cases of economic hardship

6. Establishment of an emergency transport plan with the family and the appropriate local transport team

Nursing Assessment Each Visit

The nurse will perform physical assessment and examination to evaluate the following areas:

1. Cardiovascular: Assess heart rate, rhythm, and presence of murmur. Palpate peripheral pulses and observe for edema.

2. Respiratory: Auscultate lungs for rate, rhythm, and abnormal breath sounds. Observe the character of respiratory effort (retractions, grunting, or flaring).

3. Metabolic: Assess the newborn's temperature and intake.

4. Gastrointestinal: Assess for vomiting, frequent loose stools, and irritation of the buttocks. Weigh the newborn, measure girth, and auscultate bowel sounds.

5. Genitourinary: Determine the number of wet diapers per 24 hours.

6. Musculoskeletal: Check muscle tone, vigor of activity, and movement of all extremities.

7. Neurologic: Assess the fontanel, irritability, cry, presence of jitters, and seizure activity.

8. Measure the head circumference and length weekly and plot them on the growth chart.

9. Check the newborn's weight each visit and plot it on the growth chart.

Activity

1. The newborn should be held during feedings, not propped up with a bottle.

2. At times other than feeding, provide activity appropriate to the developmental stage.

3. Provide adequate rest periods on a consistent schedule.

Diet

Review intake amounts, type of food, and frequency of feeding.

Education

1. Safety

    a. Review newborn safety; identify and correct hazards in the home.

    b. Review the signs of infection and feeding intolerance with the parents.

2. Growth and development

    a. Review development, instructing the parents in newborn stimulation, stressing the need to include tactile stimulation at times other than feeding and toys appropriate for age.

    b. Reinforce the newborn's need for a quiet, nonthreatening, and nurturing environment.

3. Rest

    a. Review the need to provide a consistent rest schedule in a quiet environment.

    b. The newborn needs to be warm and dry.

4. Miscellaneous

    a. Inform the parents of available community resources.

    b. Reinforce the need for follow-up care and immunizations.

HOME CARE PROTOCOL: FIBEROPTIC HOME PHOTOTHERAPY

Phototherapy will be initiated per order in accordance with agency general admission criteria and the criteria below.

Eligibility Requirements

1. The pediatric health care provider must refer the patient to the phototherapy program with a diagnosis of idiopathic neonatal hyperbilirubinemia.

2. The newborn must meet the following criteria:

   a. The newborn's birth weight must be over 2270 grams.

   b. The newborn must be term (37 to 40 weeks).

   c. Apgar scores should be above 7.

   d. Only vigorous, active newborns will be admitted to the program.

   e. The newborn must be feeding without difficulty.

   f. There should be adequate stooling and urination within 24 hours of birth.

   g. The newborn blood levels should be as follows:

      1) Combs test: negative

      2) Rh-sensitization: negative

      3) ABO incompatibility: negative (an ABO incompatibility in which bilirubin level is trending downward will be considered for admission; the infant's hemoglobin level must be known)

      4) Direct bilirubin: <1.5 mg/100 ml

      5) Hematocrit: less than 65%

      6) Total bilirubin level within the previous 6 hours

      7) Maternal and infant blood types must be known.

   h. The history of bilirubin level at various ages should be known (this is a guideline only).

      1) At 24 hours old, below 10 mg/100 ml

      2) At 48 hours old, below 15 mg/100 ml

      3) At 72 hours old or older, below 18 mg/100 ml

3. There should be no educational or language barriers with the parents.

4. The newborn should have an adequate home environment (there should be electricity, heat, and phone).

5. Plan for follow-up bilirubin levels daily or twice daily, depending on the orders.

6. The parents should be aware of their 24-hour monitoring responsibility.

Equipment Needed

1. Home phototherapy blanket unit containing illuminator, fiberoptic cable and panel, and disposable panel covers

2. Thermometer

3. Equipment for drawing blood samples

4. Phototherapy chart packet

    a. Parent information sheet

    b. Consent form/initial evaluation chart

    c. Nursing progress/Plan of Care

    d. Parent's record of phototherapy treatment

    e. Discharge summary

5. Three-prong grounded plug adapter

Procedure

1. Wash your hands and complete the infant assessment.

2. Provide the parents with the parent information sheet and review the family teaching flow-sheet.

3. The illuminator box should be placed only on a hard, flat surface, no more than 4 feet from where the baby will be lying or held. Be sure that the air vent in the rear of the unit is not blocked. Do not put the illuminator next to or on a radiator or heater.

4. Insert the metal collar of the fiberoptic panel completely into the insert of the illuminator. The end of the metal collar of the fiberoptic panel is designed to be even with the end of the insert of the illuminator. Turn the metal collar of the panel clockwise, one quarter-turn, to lock it in place.

5. Plug the illuminator box into an electrical outlet. You will need a three-prong plug (grounded) outlet close by for the electrical cord. A heavy-duty extension cord, such as those used for power tools or appliances, can be used.

6. Insert the panel into a disposable panel cover, ensuring that the light faces the fabric side of the cover, not the plastic side.

7. Place the covered panel around the baby, under his or her arms. Be sure that the fabric side goes against the skin. The lower part of the panel will be on the outside of the baby's diaper. Be sure the diaper is folded down below the baby's navel in front and as far as possible in the back so that as much of the skin as possible is exposed to the light.

8. Using two of the tape tabs provided, fasten the panel in place by affixing the tabs on the plastic side of the cover at the open end close to where you inserted the fiberoptic panel. You should be able to insert two fingers between the panel and the baby's skin if applied properly.

9. You can now place a T-shirt on the baby, and wrap him or her in a blanket or a sleeper. In larger or more active babies, to prevent possible skin irritation under the baby's arms, tuck a little of the baby's T-shirt, blanket, or sleeper into the top of the panel. Doing this will help cushion the infant's armpit area, preventing skin irritation.

10. Turn on the illuminator and start therapy.

11. Inform the parents of the follow-up visit plan.

12. Return for bilirubin draws as per pediatric care provider orders and deliver to the preidentified laboratory.

13. Notify the home care agency office (or the on-call supervisor) of the estimated time the lab report will be available; provide the names and phone numbers of the pediatric care provider and the laboratory.

14. The home care nurse (or the on-call supervisor) is responsible for obtaining the lab result, contacting the pediatric care provider, and coordinating the plan for further orders.

■ HOME CARE PROTOCOL: OXYGEN-DEPENDENT NEONATES

Eligibility Requirements

1. The initial acute treatment has been completed.

2. Laboratory test values are within the normal range.

3. The newborn is free of infection.

4. A pneumogram and other pertinent neonatal testing has been completed.

5. The parents have completed instruction in CPR.

6. The parents have completed instruction for oxygen administration and care of the equipment.

7. The parents have demonstrated the ability and willingness to maintain the newborn at home on oxygen.

8. The infant is taking adequate formula to promote a weight gain of 15 to 20 grams per 24 hours.

9. A pediatric care provider has been selected.

10. The predischarge assessment of the home has been completed.

11. All of the necessary equipment has been ordered.

12. The child has been discharged 24 to 48 hours after meeting the discharge criteria.

13. The electric company has been notified of the medical need for power priority.

14. The appropriate utilities have been notified of the need for water, phone, electricity, and heat in cases of economic hardship.

15. An emergency transport plan is in place.

General Nursing and Pediatric Care Provider Treatment Orders

Before discharge of the newborn from the hospital, a predischarge evaluation is to be completed. The Home Needs Assessment Tool found in the Appendices can be used for this purpose. This assessment entails the following:

1. Socioeconomic evaluation

2. Laboratory test results

3. Neonatal testing results

4. Complete physical assessment to include the following:

    a. Pertinent past and current findings

    b. Appropriate identifying information

        1) Newborn's name, address, phone number

        2) Parents' names

        3) Referring pediatric care provider's name, address, phone number

        4) Insurance type and numbers

        5) Type of home care, visits, and frequency

    c. Medications and dietary/treatment orders

    d. Assurance that the supplies and equipment needed have been ordered and that delivery has been arranged with the parents

    e. Evaluation of initial visit, establishing long-term and short-term goals

    f. Signature of the pediatric nurse and date the predischarge assessment was rendered

4. Notification of the electric company of medical priority for any child using medical electrical equipment in case of power outage

5. Notification of the appropriate utilities of need for water, phone, electricity, and heat in cases of economic hardship

6. Establishment of an emergency transport plan with the family and the appropriate local transport team

Nursing Assessment Each Visit

The nurse will perform physical assessment and examination to evaluate the following areas:

1. Cardiovascular: Assess heart rate, rhythm, and presence of murmur. Palpate peripheral pulses and observe for edema.

2. Respiratory: Auscultate breath sounds; note rate and rhythm of respiration and character of respiratory effort. Note the color of oral mucosa and nail beds. Note the flow rate and concentration of oxygen in use. Assure that nares are free of secretions that impede oxygen delivery. Follow pulse oximetry readings with the pediatric care provider and respiratory care company on the scheduled routine, per pediatric care provider orders.

3. Metabolic: Assess the newborn's temperature and intake.

4. Gastrointestinal: Assess for vomiting, frequent loose stools, and irritation of buttocks. Weigh the newborn, measure girth, and auscultate bowel sounds.

5. Genitourinary: Determine the number of wet diapers per 24 hours.

6. Musculoskeletal: Check muscle tone, vigor of activity, and movement of all extremities.

7. Neurologic: Assess the fontanel, irritability, cry, moro reflex, presence of jitters, and seizure activity.

8. Infectious disease: Note the presence/absence of upper respiratory infection.

9. Skin: Assess the skin for any evidence of breakdown.

10. Psychological: Encourage and support the parents. Assess the need for respite care.

11. Check length and head circumference each week and plot on the growth chart at least monthly.

12. Check weight at each visit and plot on the growth chart at least monthly.

Activity

1. Activity and bonding should be appropriate to age and development.

2. Avoid overstimulation that would lead to increased oxygen consumption.

3. Provide adequate rest periods.

4. Avoid prolonged exposure to outdoors during extreme cold weather, excessive heat and humidity, and inclement weather.

Diet

1. The formula type and amount will be accurately calculated and monitored if the newborn has problems with fluid retention or poor weight gain.

2. Introduction of solid foods will be supervised by the pediatric care provider.

3. Observe for allergy and note any sensitivity.

Education

1. Safety
   a. Review infant safety; identify and correct hazards in the home.
   b. Review and stress oxygen safety in the home with respect to open flame.
   c. No smoking is permissible in the presence of oxygen (oxygen supports combustion).

2. Respiratory
   a. Review chest physiotherapy and suctioning.
   b. Avoid contact between the newborn and persons with an infectious disease.
   c. Caution the parents against weaning the newborn without the doctor's orders.
   d. Review the signs of illness and feeding intolerance so parents can notify the pediatric care provider.
   e. Review the signs of respiratory distress so the parents can notify the pediatric care provider.
   f. Review the importance of a smoke-free environment.

3. Growth and development

   a. Review newborn development and stimulation to promote growth.

   b. Reinforce the need for immunizations and follow-up visits.

4. Medications

   a. Educate the family concerning the signs and symptoms of adverse reactions to medications prescribed.

   b. Observe drug levels. The newborn must have the influenza vaccine; the family must contact nurses.

5. Equipment

   a. Review the care and cleaning of the respiratory equipment.

   b. Review the use of the equipment.

6. Family support

   a. Inform the family of the available community support and assist them with referrals.

   b. Determine the need for respite care in the home by an RN or LPN.

7. Discuss with the parents the pediatric care provider's plan for weaning.

8. Discuss practical problems and appropriate solutions, problem solving, and weaning protocols. Act as a liaison between the family and pediatric care provider if indicated.

Nursing Visit Plan

Nursing visits will be conducted per the pediatric care provider's Plan of Care.

■ HOME CARE PROTOCOL: SEIZURE DISORDERS (BIRTH TO SIX MONTHS)

Eligibility Requirements

1. The initial acute treatment has been completed.

2. Laboratory test values are within the normal range.

3. The newborn is free of infection.

4. Seizures are controlled; if the newborn is on medication, side effects are minimal.

5. The parents are able to describe and recognize seizure activity and demonstrate the appropriate care.

6. The predischarge assessment in the home has been completed.

7. A pediatric care provider has been selected for follow-up care.

8. The newborn is taking adequate nutrition for weight gain of 15 to 20 grams per 24 hours on average.

9. The newborn has been discharged 24 to 48 hours after meeting the discharge criteria.

10. The electric company has been notified of the medical need for power priority.

11. The appropriate utilities have been notified of the need for water, phone, electricity, and heat in cases of economic hardship.

12. An emergency transport plan is in place.

General Nursing and Pediatric Care Provider Treatment Orders

Before discharge of the newborn from the hospital, a predischarge evaluation is to be completed. The Home Needs Assessment Tool found in the appendices can be used for this purpose. This evaluation entails the following:

1. Socioeconomic evaluation

2. Laboratory tests; medication blood levels where appropriate

3. EEG, head scan or MRI, CAT scan, and pneumogram results where appropriate

4. Complete physical assessment and history to include the following:

    a. Pertinent past and current findings, including prenatal history and neonatal course

    b. Appropriate identifying information

        1) Newborn's name, address, phone number

        2) Parents' names

        3) Referring pediatric care provider's name, address, phone number

       4) Insurance type and numbers

       5) Type of home care, visits, and frequency

    c. Medications, dietary plans, and activity level

    d. Supplies and equipment needed

    e. Evaluation of initial visit, establishing long-term and short-term goals

    f. Signature of the pediatric nurse and date the predischarge assessment was rendered

5. Notification of the electric company of medical priority for any newborn using medical electrical equipment in case of a power outage

6. Notification of the appropriate utilities of the need for water, phone, electricity, and heat in cases of economic hardship

7. Establishment of an emergency transport plan with the family and the appropriate local transport team

Nursing Assessment Each Visit

The nurse will perform physical assessment and examination to evaluate the following areas:

1. Cardiovascular: Assess heart rate, rhythm, and presence of murmur. Palpate peripheral pulses and observe for edema. Assess skin color.

2. Respiratory: Auscultate lungs for rate, rhythm, and abnormal breath sounds. Observe the character of respiratory effort (retractions, grunting, or flaring).

3. Metabolic: Assess the newborn's temperature and intake.

4. Gastrointestinal: Assess for vomiting, frequent loose stools, and irritation of buttocks. Weigh the newborn, measure girth, and auscultate bowel sounds.

5. Genitourinary: Determine the number of wet diapers per 24 hours.

6. Musculoskeletal: Check muscle tone, vigor of activity, and movement of all extremities.

7. Neurologic: Assess responsiveness and level of consciousness. Observe for presence of shunt and signs of irritation along shunt. Determine if the newborn has been vomiting or is irritable or lethargic. Assess for sunset eyes and check pupillary reaction to light. Check for signs of intracranial pressure by assessing the newborn's cry, posture, fontanel, and head circumference.

8. Psychological: Encourage and support the family. Allow them to express their feelings or ask questions.

Activity

1. The newborn should be treated as normally as possible with play activities and newborn stimulation appropriate for age and development.

2. Avoid excess fatigue and exhaustion.

3. Pad the sides of the crib and the playpen to protect the newborn.

Diet

1. There are no dietary restrictions.

2. Avoid excessive intake of water or other hypotonic fluids.

Education

1. Identification of seizures
    a. Explain the specific cause for the seizure.
    b. Explain the significance of seizures (what effect they have on brain function).

2. Safety
    a. Review newborn safety; identify and correct hazards in the home.
    b. Reinforce the need to pad the sides of the crib or playpen.

3. Medications
    a. Minimize the side effects of antiepileptic drug therapy.
    b. Reinforce the necessity of giving medications at the same time daily and at the correct dosage. Never miss a dose.
    c. Review the actions of drugs and adverse reactions, which should be reported if observed.
    d. Review any known drug allergies of the newborn with the parents as well as information about any other medications the newborn is receiving.

4. Growth and development
    a. Review newborn development and stimulation to promote growth.
    b. Reinforce the need for immunizations and follow-up visits.
    c. Provide a daily gum massage for a newborn on Dilantin.

5. In the following situations, notify the pediatric care provider and care for the newborn as described below:
    a. Development of fever, nausea, vomiting, and diarrhea will affect the metabolism of pharmaceutical agents and/or may lead to increased seizure activity.
    b. For a temperature higher than 101°F, instruct the parents to give acetaminophen and a lukewarm sponge bath.
    c. Increased seizure activity without illness requires notification of the pediatric care provider because the newborn's doses may need to be adjusted for growth.

6. Supportive help
    a. Inform the parents of the available community resources and assist them in obtaining help.
    b. When the newborn has a seizure, remain calm and stay with the newborn. The seizure cannot be stopped once it has begun. Place the newborn on a flat cushioned surface or hold him or her gently. Do not restrain the newborn. Clear the area of objects that may injure the newborn. Maintain a patent airway. Provide time for recovery after the seizure stops. Reassure and provide support for the newborn and others.

■ HOME CARE PROTOCOL: THE CHILD WITH A COLOSTOMY

Eligibility Requirements

1. The initial acute treatment has been completed.

2. Laboratory test values are within the normal range.

3. The newborn is free of infection.

4. The newborn is gaining weight at a rate of 15 to 20 grams per 24 hours on average.

5. A discharge diet plan has been completed.

6. Parents have received instruction in care of a colostomy.

7. A pediatric care provider has been selected for follow-up care.

8. The predischarge assessment in the home has been completed.

9. Colostomy care equipment has been ordered.

10. The newborn has been discharged 24 to 48 hours after meeting the discharge criteria.

11. The electric company has been notified of the medical need for power priority.

12. The appropriate utilities have been notified of need for water, phone, electricity, and heat in cases of economic hardship.

13. An emergency transport plan is in place.

General Nursing and Pediatric Care Provider Treatment Orders

Before discharge of the newborn from the hospital, a predischarge evaluation is to be completed. The Home Needs Assessment Tool found in the Appendices can be used for this purpose. The assessment entails the following:

1. Socioeconomic evaluation

2. Laboratory tests

3. Neonatal testing results, including pneumogram results where appropriate

4. Complete a physical assessment and history to include the following:
   a. Pertinent past and current findings, including birth history and hospital course
   b. Appropriate identifying information
      1) Newborn's name, address, phone number
      2) Parents' names
      3) Referring pediatric care provider's name, address, phone number

        4) Insurance type and numbers

        5) Type of home care, visits, and frequency

    c. Medications, dietary plans, and activity

    d. Supplies and equipment needed

    e. Evaluation of initial visit, establishing long-term and short-term goals

    f. Signature of the pediatric nurse and date the predischarge assessment was rendered

5. Notification of the electric company of medical priority for any child using medical electrical equipment in case of a power outage

6. Notification of the appropriate utilities of the need for water, phone, electricity, and heat in cases of economic hardship

7. Establishment of an emergency transport plan with the family and the appropriate local transport team

Nursing Assessment Each Visit

1. The nurse will perform physical assessment and examination to evaluate the following:

    a. Cardiovascular: Auscultate heart rate and rhythm; assess for murmur; palpate pulses and note edema.

    b. Respiratory: Auscultate breath sounds, note abnormal breath sounds; observe for rate, rhythm, and character of respirations.

    c. Metabolic: Assess the newborn's temperature and test the urine for glucose and protein.

    d. Gastrointestinal: Assess for vomiting, characteristics of stool, and appearance of skin around stoma. Check the newborn's weight; check the stool for blood and reducing substance. Review intake with the parents. Auscultate bowel sounds.

    e. Genitourinary: Check the number of wet diapers; observe for fluid retention.

    f. Musculoskeletal: Observe for activity and equal movement of all extremities. Note any abnormal markings on the body.

    g. Neurologic: Palpate fontanels; check moro reflex, hyper- or hypotonicity of extremities. Note the quality of the cry and sucking ability.

2. Assess parent–newborn attachment and interaction, identifying potential and existing problems.

Activity

Determine that the newborn in the home environment is engaged in activity appropriate for developmental and chronological stage.

Diet

The formula type and volume will be determined by the pediatric care provider.

Education

Instruct the family about feedings.

1. Review the importance of good nutrition.

2. Increase the amount of formula per hunger and growth.

3. Review the signs of feeding intolerance.

Safety

Review newborn safety; identify and correct hazards in the home.

Colostomy Care

1. Outline all the equipment needs and breakdown of the stoma.

2. Reinforce the need to keep the skin clean around the stoma.

3. Observe the parents changing the bag; offer assistance as needed.

Growth and Development

Review activities appropriate for newborn stimulation and normal growth and development.

■ HOME CARE PROTOCOL: TRACHEOSTOMY IN THE NEONATE WITH CHRONIC LUNG DISEASE

Eligibility Requirements

1. The initial acute treatment has been completed.

2. Laboratory test values are within the normal limits.

3. The newborn is free of infection.

4. A pneumogram and other pertinent neonatal tests have been completed.

5. The need for an apnea bradycardia monitor has been determined.

6. The parents have been instructed in CPR.

7. Instruction in tracheostomy care and suctioning has been completed.

8. The infant is taking formula to promote a weight gain of 15 to 20 grams per 24 hours on average.

9. A pediatric care provider has been selected for follow-up care.

10. The predischarge assessment of the home has been completed.

11. All of the necessary equipment has been ordered.

12. The newborn has been discharged 24 to 48 hours after meeting the discharge criteria.

13. The electric company has been notified of the medical need for power priority.

14. The appropriate utilities have been notified of the need for water, phone, electricity, and heat in cases of economic hardship.

15. An emergency transport plan is in place.

General Nursing and Pediatric Care Provider Treatment Orders

Before discharge of the newborn from the hospital, a predischarge evaluation is to be completed. A home assessment should be performed. The Home Needs Assessment Tool found in the Appendices can be used for this purpose. The assessment entails the following:

1. Socioeconomic evaluation

2. Laboratory tests

3. Neonatal testing results

4. Complete physical assessment and history to include the following:
   a. Birth history and hospital course

    b. Appropriate identifying information

       1) Newborn's name, address, phone number

       2) Parents' names

       3) Referring pediatric care provider's name, address, phone number

       4) Insurance type and numbers

       5) Type of home care, visits, and frequency

    c. Medications and dietary/treatment orders

    d. Supplies and equipment needed

    e. Evaluation of initial visit, establishing long-term and short-term goals

    f. Signature of the pediatric nurse and date the predischarge assessment was rendered

5. Notification of the electric company of medical priority for any newborn using medical electrical equipment in case of a power outage

6. Notification of the appropriate utilities of the need for water, phone, electricity, and heat in cases of economic hardship

7. Establishment of an emergency transport plan with the family and the appropriate local transport team

Nursing Assessment Each Visit

The nurse will perform physical assessment and examination to evaluate the following:

1. Cardiovascular: Assess heart rate, rhythm, and presence of murmur. Palpate peripheral pulses and observe for edema.

2. Respiratory: Auscultate breath sounds for wheezing and air entry. Assess for bronchospasm; suction if necessary. Observe rate, rhythm, and character of respiration. Note the appropriate use of oxygen; assess the tracheostomy site for breakdown.

3. Metabolic: Assess the newborn's temperature and intake.

4. Gastrointestinal: Assess for vomiting, frequent loose stools, and irritation of buttocks. Weigh the newborn, measure girth, and auscultate bowel sounds.

5. Genitourinary: Determine the number of wet diapers per 24 hours.

6. Musculoskeletal: Check muscle tone, vigor of activity, and movement of all extremities.

7. Neurologic: Assess the fontanel, irritability, cry, presence of jitters, seizure activity, and movement of all extremities.

Activity

1. Feed the newborn in a comfortable position at a 30° to 45° angle.

2. Activity should be appropriate to age and development, with adequate rest periods.

Diet

The diet will be ordered by the pediatric care provider.

Education

1. Safety

    a. Review newborn safety; identify and correct hazards in the home.

    b. Toys

        1) Avoid toys with small removable parts.

        2) Avoid stuffed animals and furry toys.

        3) Instruct parents not to allow the newborn to put toys, food, or other small objects into the tracheostomy tube.

    c. Feeding

        1) Prevent food from entering tracheostomy by using a bib (placed loosely to avoid occlusion).

        2) Position the newborn on his or her side after eating to prevent aspiration.

    d. Environment

        1) Stay with the newborn during bathing or playing in a wading pool. A humidity collar or humidivent can be used to protect the tracheostomy from water splashes.

        2) Protect the newborn from irritants (hair sprays, talcum powders, perfume, smoke, ammonia products, pet hairs).

        3) Avoid exposure to extremely cold air (which causes tracheal spasm) and dust particles. The tracheostomy can be loosely covered on extremely cold, windy, or dusty days.

    e. Clothing

        1) Keep clothing away from the airway.

        2) A light covering may be used to prevent extreme cold, irritants, food, or dust entering the tracheostomy.

2. Respiratory

    a. Assess respiratory status. Instruct the family about the signs and symptoms of respiratory distress.

    b. Review the necessity of having an extra tracheostomy tube, ties, and emergency equipment at the bedside and available at all times.

    c. Review the signs of an obstructed airway and ways to correct the problem.

    d. Review chest physiotherapy technique and care of the tracheostomy.

    e. Reinforce the appropriate technique for suctioning; observe the amount, color, and odor of tracheostomy secretions.

    f. Observe and reinforce the technique for changing the tracheostomy tube and tracheostomy ties. Two people are required to change the ties.

    g. Review the need to provide humidification to prevent drying of tissues and to loosen secretions.

   h. Reinforce the need to avoid contact between the newborn and infectious persons.

   i. Praise the family in their care of the newborn.

3. Growth and development

   a. Review newborn development and the need for stimulation to promote adequate growth and development.

   b. Reinforce the need for immunizations and follow-up visits.

4. Medications

   a. If drug levels are to be monitored, assist in obtaining necessary specimens.

   b. Instruct the family on medication administration technique, dosage, action, and side effects.

   c. Instruct the family on adverse reactions to medications that should be reported to the pediatric care provider.

5. Equipment: Ensure that the family can competently operate and clean the necessary equipment.

6. Support services: Coordinate and supervise physical therapy, occupational therapy, speech therapy, and the medical social worker if ordered.

7. Miscellaneous

   a. Inform the parents of community resources available.

   b. Review measures for minimizing irritability.

■ HOME CARE PROTOCOL: CYSTIC FIBROSIS

Eligibility Requirements

1. Acute exacerbation of the disease has occurred, or a new diagnosis of the disease has been made.

2. Laboratory test values are at an acceptable, manageable level.

3. The newborn is free of infection or the infection is being controlled with oral antibiotics.

4. Parents have received instruction in the following areas:

    a. Chest physiotherapy and postural drainage

    b. Dietary treatment plans

    c. Medication administration

    d. Use of oxygen, aerosol treatments, and vaporizer

    e. Interventions indicated during a crisis

5. A social service evaluation has been completed.

6. A pediatric care provider has been selected for follow-up care.

7. A dietary plan for discharge has been prepared.

8. A predischarge assessment in the home has been completed.

9. All of the necessary equipment has been ordered.

10. The patient has been discharged 24 to 48 hours after meeting the discharge criteria.

11. The electric company has been notified of the medical need for power priority.

12. The appropriate utilities have been notified of the need for water, phone, electricity, and heat in cases of economic hardship.

13. An emergency transport plan is in place.

General Nursing and Pediatric Care Provider Treatment Orders

Before discharge of the newborn from the hospital, a predischarge evaluation is to be completed. The Home Needs Assessment Tool found in the Appendices can be used for this purpose. This assessment entails:

1. Socioeconomic evaluation

2. Laboratory tests

3. Pediatric testing results

4. Complete physical assessment and history to include the following information:

    a. Birth history and hospital course

    b. Appropriate identifying information

       1) Newborn's name, address, phone number

       2) Parents' names

       3) Referring pediatric care provider's name, address, phone number

       4) Insurance type and numbers

       5) Type of home care, visits, and frequency

    c. Medications and dietary/treatment orders

    d. Supplies and equipment needed

    e. Evaluation of initial visit, establishing long-term and short-term goals

    f. Signature of the pediatric nurse and date the predischarge assessment was rendered

5. Notification of the electric company of medical priority for any newborn using medical electrical equipment in case of a power outage

6. Notification of the appropriate utilities of the need for water, phone, electricity, and heat in cases of economic hardship

7. Establishment of an emergency transport plan with the family and the appropriate local transport team

Nursing Assessment Each Visit

The nurse will perform physical assessment and examination to evaluate the following areas:

1. Cardiovascular: Assess the heart rate, rhythm, and presence of murmur. Palpate peripheral pulses and observe for edema.

2. Respiratory: Auscultate breath sounds for equal air entry and abnormal sounds. Note rate, rhythm, and degree of respiratory effort. Observe for dyspnea, tachypnea, retractions, flaring, and cyanosis of oral mucosa and nail beds. Note the presence of cough and production of secretions. Review appropriate oxygen use if indicated.

3. Metabolic: Assess oral temperature. Palpate skin to determine if it is warm and dry or cool and clammy. Obtain a detailed account of the newborn's dietary intake from the parents, including the volume of fluids.

4. Gastrointestinal: Assess for vomiting, nausea, and diarrhea. If stool is available during the visit, note the color, character, and frequency. Weigh the newborn; auscultate bowel sounds.

5. Genitourinary: Note output.

6. Musculoskeletal: Assess muscle tone, skin turgor, and ability to move all extremities.

7. Neurologic: Assess pupil reaction and presence of irritability.

8. Psychological: Assess the family's acceptance and handling of the disease. Support the family.

Activity

1. The infant may attend day care between exacerbations of the disease.

2. The infant may engage in play appropriate for his or her age, as tolerated between exacerbations and dyspnea. Play should be of a more sedentary nature when recovering from exacerbations.

3. Assist the parents in finding diversionary activities while the newborn is recuperating at home.

Diet

Adequate nutrition is necessary for growth and development.

1. The diet should be high in calories, high in protein, and low in fat.

2. Water-soluble vitamins should be given in doses 2 to 3 times the normal dosage.

3. Absent pancreatic enzymes should be replaced with extracts of animal pancreas. Give with each meal.

4. Salt intake should be increased during hot weather or excessive exercise.

5. Caregivers should be patient with the newborn during feeding.

Education

1. Safety
    a. Review newborn safety; identify and correct hazards in the home.
    b. Review oxygen safety if oxygen is being used in the home.

2. Medications
    a. Review desired effects of and adverse reactions to the prescribed medications.
    b. Emphasize the importance of administering vitamins and enzymes regularly and of not missing a dose.

▦ HOME CARE PROTOCOL: EDUCATING PARENTS/CAREGIVERS ABOUT DIARRHEA AND NUTRITION

The major complication from gastroenteritis is dehydration and accompanying electrolyte imbalance. Signs of dehydration may not always be apparent to parents. Parents should be informed of these signs and should report them. Assessment data provide the basis for decision making pertaining to treatment and care concerning infant diarrhea and nutrition. One-to-one teaching that is culturally sensitive and that uses language the caregiver can easily understand is the goal.

Criteria

Home visits are recommended in cases of infants presenting to the emergency room with the following conditions.

1. Acute gastroenteritis (AGE)

2. Vomiting (with no evidence of intestinal obstruction or acute abdomen)

3. Poor intake

4. Dehydration (excluding those patients exhibiting signs of circulatory collapse)

Recommended Visit Pattern

Daily visits are suggested to monitor intake, output, and daily weight; to provide physical assessments; and to ensure compliance with the treatment regime.

▦ PARENT EDUCATION PROGRAM: DIARRHEA

Diarrhea is one of the most common problems in infants, as well as one of the most potentially dangerous. The following information should be helpful in understanding exactly what is going on in the child's body, how to treat diarrhea, and how not to treat diarrhea.

Diarrhea and Dehydration

1. Definition of diarrhea: Three or more liquid stools (liquid bowel movements) in a day.

2. Causes of diarrhea
   a. Germs, bacterial or viral, that cause an infection of the intestines (bowels). This is called gastroenteritis.
   b. Microscopic animal organisms. Giardia is a common cause of a highly contagious diarrhea often transmitted from infant to infant in day care centers.
   c. Fungus (candida is one species) can cause diarrhea, especially in infants who have been weakened by other illnesses or who have immune-deficiency diseases.

    d. Parasitic worms are very common among infants, who tend to put their unwashed fingers and hands in or near their mouths.

    e. Physiologic causes include fever. Many infants get diarrhea along with a cold, change in diet, milk intolerance, or rich or spicy foods.

Regardless of the cause, diarrhea should stop within a week. If it continues, call the infant's doctor or clinic.

3. Impact of diarrhea on the infant's health

    a. Colds and diarrhea are the two most common illnesses of infants. Worldwide, infants have 1 to 10 episodes of diarrhea a year.

    b. Diarrhea can cause dehydration from fluid loss.

    c. Common diarrhea can cause serious illness or even death, especially in very young infants. In the United States, 200,000 infants per year are hospitalized and 500 infants die as a result of dehydration from diarrhea. This can be prevented if pediatric care providers and caregivers understand diarrhea, dehydration, and simple steps they can take to prevent them.

4. Definition/explanation of dehydration

    a. At birth, the human body is about 80% water. By 9 months, it is 60% water and should stay at that level.

    b. Electrolytes are special kinds of salts (sodium and potassium) in the body that are vital to the body's systems.

    c. Diarrhea causes body fluids and electrolytes to be lost in the stool. This can cause dehydration and even death.

5. Signs of dehydration (indicating a lack of fluid)

    a. Dry mouth (lips or tongue)

    b. Unusual drowsiness, listlessness, or fussiness

    c. Extreme thirst

    d. Sunken-looking eyes

    e. Decreased urination (or less than six wet diapers per day or a period of longer than 4 hours without urination)

    f. Concentrated urine (urine is very dark yellow)

    g. Absence of tears

    h. Rapid heartbeat or pulse

    i. Sunken soft spot (fontanel)

    j. Poor skin turgor (pinch skin on abdomen; the skin should return to normal after being released)

6. What to do if an infant is dehydrated.

    a. If an infant with diarrhea appears dehydrated, has a fever over 101°, cannot drink fluids, or has blood in the stool, call a doctor or clinic ***immediately***. Blood in the stool can make it look red, rust-colored, or flecked with blood.

    b. ***If an infant with diarrhea is unconscious, "floppy," or has a high fever (more than 103°), take the infant immediately to the nearest hospital!***

7. Management of gastroenteritis involves three components.

   a. Maintain or restore fluid and electrolyte balance.

   b. Restore the bowel to normal functioning.

   c. Prevent the infection of others in contact with the infant.

8. Care of an infant with diarrhea
   These guidelines will help you to help your infant get well, keep him or her out of the hospital, and avoid a painful needle stick for intravenous treatment.

   a. Rehydration
      To prevent and treat dehydration, start oral rehydration therapy (ORT) as soon as the diarrhea begins. ORT is discussed and explained in detail in the next section.

   b. Feeding

      1) Sometimes people think that it is necessary to "rest the gut" in cases of diarrhea. ***This is not a good practice!*** It is very important that infants eat when they are sick, even when they have diarrhea. Eating the right foods actually helps the infant get well faster. The right foods give the infant the energy needed for healing and for fighting the infection causing the diarrhea. Small, frequent feedings are most often given, yet larger quantities offered less frequently may be recommended because frequent feedings have the potential to induce peristalsis.

      2) ***DO continue to breastfeed or bottlefeed your baby normally*** (unless instructed otherwise by your baby's pediatric care provider).

      3) ***DO NOT give the infant sugary or salty foods or drinks.*** These can make the diarrhea worse.

9. Medication for diarrhea
   Diarrhea is a reaction of the intestines to an infection or irritation. The very best care for most cases of infant diarrhea is simply replacing the fluids and salts lost by giving oral rehydration solution and feeding the infant good foods while he or she is sick or following an illness.

   Parents are usually very concerned about the frequency and appearance of bowel movements and want to give the infant something to "bind" the bowels. This does not really help because, when the infant has diarrhea, the body fluid and salts are still being lost. They are just being held in the intestine longer. The fluid in the intestine does not go back into the body where it is needed! It is possible that the infant is still becoming dehydrated, even though the diarrheal bowel movements are not being expelled. So, "binding" the infant will give parents a false sense of security because it appears that the diarrhea is getting better. It is not—it is just being held inside longer. Also, you might not realize how much fluid is being lost because it is "hidden" in the intestine, so you will not realize how much the infant needs to drink.

   Remember, the main goal is to prevent dehydration and to recognize it early if it does develop.

10. Record keeping
    If your infant has diarrhea it may be helpful to keep a written record, so that if you have to call the pediatric care provider you will be prepared to ask and answer questions. Start the notes as soon as the diarrhea starts. You should record the following information.

    a. Amount and color of the stool and time

    b. Amount and kind of fluid the infant takes and time

    c. Temperature

    d. Weight

If you have a scale, weigh the infant as soon as the diarrhea starts, especially if the infant is under 3 years old. If you have this information when you need to call the doctor, nurse, or clinic, they will be able to decide more easily if the infant should be brought in.

11. Comfort the infant
    Infants with diarrhea do not feel well and therefore have special needs. Babies' bottoms hurt and they may be cranky. These are some things you can do to prevent and treat diaper rash to make the baby feel better.

    a. Do not use baby wipes that contain alcohol.

    b. Do change diapers often.

    c. Do wash the infant's bottom with soap, rinse with plain warm water, and gently pat dry.

    d. Do apply Vaseline, Desitin, or A&D ointment to the infant's bottom. This will keep the stool away from the skin.

    e. Do apply cornstarch or baby powder to the infant's bottom.

12. Prevention of diarrhea
    The microorganisms (germs) that cause diarrhea are passed by people, objects, and food. To prevent the spread of diarrhea, here are some things you can do.

    a. Wash your hands well with soap and water.

        1) Before cooking food or feeding your infant

        2) After changing your infant's diaper or going to the toilet

        3) After handling raw meat of any kind

        4) After giving a sick infant medication or feeding

    b. Do not let infants play with, or put into their mouths, things that you know are dirty.

    c. Throw disposable diapers out immediately and keep them in a trash can away from infants and pets. The trash can should have a lid.

    d. Keep dirty cloth diapers away from infants and pets and wash them as soon as possible.

    e. Be careful how you store and prepare foods. To prevent the spread of diarrhea from food, be sure to cook and prepare foods correctly and wash dishes and utensils well after use. Foods to be especially careful with are eggs, fish and shellfish, chicken, and pork. Promptly refrigerate foods that can spoil.

Oral Rehydration Therapy (ORT)

1. Definition: Oral rehydration therapy involves drinking a special solution to replace, in the proper proportions, essential body fluids and salts lost during diarrhea to treat and ***prevent dehydration***.

2. Why ORT works: The special salts (electrolytes) and water that are lost in diarrhea are needed by the body to function properly. Drinking a balanced solution of salt, water, and sugar can prevent as well as treat dehydration of people with diarrhea. These solutions are called oral rehydration solutions (ORS) or oral electrolyte solutions (OES).

3. For the solution to work best, proper amounts of the ingredients are critical. Too little or too much of any of the ingredients will cause the solution to not work correctly. (This is why an infant with diarrhea should not have salty or sugary foods and drinks and why plain water is not enough.) However, fluids are critical, and oral rehydration solution is the best replacement fluid. If ORS is not available, then any fluid is better than none.

4. Oral rehydration solutions

    a. What they are

        1) Oral rehydration solutions are special mixtures of water and electrolytes in the correct quantities that will replace the fluids and salts lost in diarrhea.

        2) Commercial brands of ORS are available, including Pedialyte, Ricelyte, and generic brands, which can be found in grocery stores and drug stores.

        3) ***There is also a solution that you can make at home*** that is a good substitute for commercial brands when it is made according to the directions. It is very ***easy*** and ***inexpensive*** to make; the recipe is provided below.

    b. How and when to give them to infants

        1) ***How*** you give the solution is as important as what you give to an infant. To prevent dehydration it is necessary to replace the fluid and salts lost in the stool, so it is important to give enough solution.

        2) When an infant has diarrhea, he or she may have an upset stomach. It is very important to give the solution slowly enough that it can be absorbed by the body and not cause the infant to vomit. Here is a general guide to giving an oral rehydration solution.

            (a) Encourage the infant to take the solution after each stool or every few minutes.

            (b) The solution should be taken in small amounts, either in sips or by spoon, so that it is easily absorbed. Do not let the infant gulp it down.

            (c) An infant under 24 months may need $1/4$ to $1/2$ cup. A child 2 to 10 years old may need $1/2$ to 1 cup.

        3) Remember, the solution is replacing what is lost in the diarrhea, so if there is a lot of diarrhea, be sure to give enough of the oral rehydration solution after each stool.

        4) If the infant vomits, keep giving the solution, but give it in sips of $1/2$ to 1 teaspoon every few minutes. This will allow time for it to be absorbed. The rate may need to be slower than before the infant vomited.

        5) When people have the correct amount of fluids and salts in their systems, they urinate often and their urine is clear to light yellow in color. If an infant's urine is dark yellow or the infant is not urinating as much as usual, you may wish to give more oral rehydration solution. Call the doctor or clinic if this condition continues.

    c. How to make homemade cereal-based ORS (the sugar is replaced in this solution by the cereal, which is a complex sugar)

        Grandma's ORS Recipe

        $1/2$ to 1 cup of precooked baby rice cereal
        2 cups of water
        $1/4$ teaspoon of table salt

        Mix all of the ingredients together until well mixed. Be sure to use a level measuring teaspoon. Make the mixture as thick as is drinkable.

Give it a little at a time, give it often, and give as much as the infant will take. (Give a little every minute if the infant will take it.) You can offer Grandma's ORS with a spoon or a cup. Remember, no gulping. Do not give too much; salt can be dangerous. Remember the idea of replacing fluid: one cup out, one cup in. In other words, the amount of diarrhea that comes out is the amount of fluid that should be put back in.

The ORS solution should be covered and stored in the refrigerator if possible. The solution should be discarded after 6 to 8 hours, or when it is too thick to drink.

Reminder: This is not considered food, and the infant should also be encouraged to eat a normal diet of breast milk, formula, and/or recommended foods.

CHAPTER 6

Family Education Materials

The teaching material found in this chapter is meant to to copied and distributed to home care nurses and the families they assist. These are only a few of the teaching tools one can access with a little research. Excellent materials can be found through The Division of Maternal Child Health, Health and Human Services (5600 Fishers Lane, Rockville, MD 20857). In addition, further resources should be available through state and local health departments. Visual and written aids assist the nurse in the education process by stimulating multiple senses and thus increasing stimulation of the memory.

Keep in mind that these items are simply *tools*. They are meant to assist in the educational process. They are not a substitute for the nurse–client relationship that develops out of a nurse's empathy with the client. The nurse should always take the time to review these handouts with clients. Do not assume the client can read or has developed an adequate trusting relationship with you to value your information. Nurses in home care work in the domain of the client, not in the office or the hospital. The nurse's ability to communicate and develop the "helping relationship" is crucial to success in providing care.

■ PARENT EDUCATION PROGRAM: POSTPARTUM INSTRUCTIONS FOR MOTHERS

Rest

1. The new mother should get plenty of rest for the first couple of weeks.

2. The client should care for herself and her baby only; she shouldn't expect too much of herself.

3. The new mother should obtain help for general household duties (cleaning, cooking, laundry, shopping, and caring for older children).

4. Emphasize that the new mother needs to rest when the baby is sleeping.

5. Limit visitors to relatives and close friends.

6. Remember, fatigue decreases the milk supply and the ability to cope with new and added responsibilities.

Activity

1. Limit stair climbing for the first week.

2. The client should let her body be the guide for activity and exercise.

3. The new mother may go out to dinner or for a ride but she should not drive for 1 to 2 weeks unless otherwise instructed by her physician. Cesarean section patients should verify with their OB care provider when driving is permitted.

Diet

1. Advise the client to drink 8 to 10 glasses of water per day.

2. Her diet should consist of protein, fruits, vegetables, and milk.

3. A small bowl of bran daily will prevent constipation

4. The client should continue taking prenatal vitamins daily at least until the postpartum exam. If the OB care provider has not instructed her to do so, the client should verify this with her physician.

5. An adequate diet as shown above is important, particularly if the mother is breastfeeding, because it takes about 800 calories daily to produce the milk the baby needs.

6. Remember, if the new mother does not eat, she will become fatigued and milk volume will decrease.

Vaginal Discharge

1. At first discharge is red, like a heavy period, for 1 to 3 days.

2. By the 3rd day the discharge should have thinned and lightened in color.

3. By the 10th day the discharge is often a pale pink, watery fluid, heavy enough to wear a light pad.

4. If, after the 3rd day, bleeding becomes bright red and heavy again, it is often a sign that the new mother has done too much and should slow down and rest.

Intercourse

1. For the majority of women, intercourse may be resumed when the vaginal area feels comfortable and the episiotomy has healed. She should check any doubts with her physician.

2. Gentleness and added lubrication may be needed for comfort when sexual activity is first resumed.

3. Breastfeeding mothers may ovulate before their first menstrual period, therefore it is possible to get pregnant again even before menstruation has resumed.

4. Foam and condoms will provide contraception if sexual activity is resumed before 6 weeks postpartum.

5. Birth control can be discussed at the 6-week postpartum visit.

Baths and Showers

1. The new mother may shower as necessary, but stress two points. ***Do not*** take a tub bath for at least 3 days unless otherwise instructed by the OB care provider. ***Do not*** use bubble bath or oils in the bath water.

2. Warm showers may help to relieve the discomfort of breast engorgement.

3. ***Do not use douches!!!***

Stitches and Hemorrhoids

1. Warm tub baths or sitz baths are recommended several times a day.

2. For discomfort of hemorrhoids use Nupercainol cream, Dermoplast, or Tucks pads. The client should consult her OB care provider.

3. There is no cause for alarm if a week or two postpartum loose stitches are found on a pad or in the toilet.

4. Reassure the new mother that stitches normally are absorbed or loosen when they no longer are needed.

Postpartum Blues

1. The new mother may experience postpartum blues during the first 10 days postpartum. The most common symptom is unexpected and unexplainable crying. Also, she may feel irritable.

2. Postpartum blues usually go away about 72 hours after onset, but they may continue for as long as 10 days.

3. If postpartum blues symptoms persist or increase in severity, they may be an early sign of postpartum depression.

4. Postpartum depression is experienced by 10% of all women and may occur anywhere within 6 months after delivery.

5. Signs and symptoms of postpartum depression
    a. Sleep disturbances may occur.
    b. Loss of appetite is common.
    c. Fear and anxiety are also signs of postpartum depression.
    d. A feeling of hopelessness may develop.
    e. Hostility or self-blame are also common.
    f. Difficulty concentrating or making decisions is another sign.

6. The client may want to seek professional help if the signs and symptoms of postpartum depression are experienced.

Baby's Fussy Periods

1. The baby may go through fussy periods during the day or evening.

2. Fussy periods may happen because the mother's milk supply is low at the end of the day.

3. The new mother may need to nurse more frequently.

4. Use calming tactics such as rocking, walking, strollers, swings, etc.

5. Lay the baby down to see if he or she will sleep.

Postpartum Problems

Call your health care provider if any of the following problems occur.

1. A flulike feeling, fever, or chills

2. A foul-smelling discharge or unusual abdominal tenderness

3. Redness and tenderness of the breasts

4. Extreme tenderness of the episiotomy area

5. Tenderness of the pubic bone, accompanied by frequency, urgency, and burning with urination

These symptoms may indicate an infection requiring professional attention and treatment.

PARENT EDUCATION PROGRAM: NEWBORN INSTRUCTIONS

Bathing

1. Sponge bathe the newborn with mild soap (low alkaline) such as Dove or Castille until the cord has fallen off and the area is completely healed.

2. Do not use oil or powder on the baby's head or skin.

3. When the navel is healed, the baby may have a tub bath.

4. Bathe the baby before feeding.

Cord Care

1. The cord usually falls off within 7 to 10 days.

2. Use alcohol and cotton to cleanse and bathe the area around the base of the cord at every diaper change.

3. There may be one or two drops of blood when the cord separates.

4. Keep the diaper folded beneath the navel to facilitate drying of the cord.

5. Call the pediatric care provider if the cord has a foul odor or if the skin of the abdominal area around the umbilical cord becomes red.

Diaper Rash

1. Change the baby's diaper when it is soiled.

2. Avoid using plastic pants when possible or change the baby frequently. Air the buttocks when changing.

3. Diapers should be washed with mild soap and rinsed well after each laundering.

4. Apply Balmex or Desitin to the diaper area, especially the creases, at each diaper change (Vaseline can be used all the time on the diaper area).

Circumcision

Apply Vaseline liberally at every diaper change until the area is no longer red or swollen.

Nails

1. Use an emery board to file nails. They are too soft to cut with scissors for the first couple of weeks.

2. Never cut with cuticle scissors

Clothing

1. Keep the baby warm, but do not overheat.

2. Use simple, easily washed clothes.

3. On hot days, a diaper and T-shirt may be enough.

4. The baby should wear one more layer of clothing than his or her mother.

5. If it is cool and breezy, the baby's head should be covered.

Feeding

1. If breastfeeding, refer to instructions and information on breastfeeding.

2. Hold the baby at every feeding.

3. Feed the baby when he or she is hungry (usually every 3 to 5 hours).

4. Do not wake the baby at night.

5. Burp the baby after every $1/2$ to 1 ounce at first.

6. Place the baby on his or her stomach or right side (roll the blanket and place behind the back for support).
   "Recent research shows that SIDS is more common in babies who go to sleep on their tummies. By making sure your baby goes to sleep on its back or side, you can help reduce the risk of SIDS" (*Back to Sleep: Reducing the Risk of Sudden Infant Death Syndrome—What You Can Do*. U.S. Public Health Service, the American Academy of Pediatrics, the SIDS Alliance, and the Association of SIDS Program Professionals). If you have any questions about your baby's sleep position, contact your health care provider first. Then you can call, toll free, 1-800-505-CRIB, or write to Back to Sleep, P.O. Box 29111, Washington DC 20040, for more information.

7. Do not start any new foods (cereal, juice, or fruit) until the pediatric care provider gives permission.

8. Use formula as ordered by the pediatric care provider. The powdered form may be more economical. The client should always follow the instructions on the can for mixing and preparing the formula.

9. The baby may have 1 to 2 ounces of boiled, cooled water if fussy.

Bowel Movements

1. The breastfed baby's bowel movements are normally loose and unformed.

2. The breastfed baby may have several small movements each day or may go for several days without having a bowel movement at all.

3. A totally breastfed baby is never constipated and seldom has diarrhea (watery bowel movements). Relax with your infant. He or she will adjust to you. If you are tense, the baby will feel tense; if you are relaxed, it will help relax your baby.

■ PARENT EDUCATION PROGRAM: BREASTFEEDING

Position for Breastfeeding

1. Assume a comfortable position (sitting, lying, football hold); positions should be rotated to avoid stress or sore nipples.

2. Bring the baby to the nipple. You may want to use pillows. This avoids the stress of the baby pulling on the nipples.

3. Expose the breast. Support the baby's head in the crook of the arm, with the other hand supporting the nipple in a scissorslike hold or thumb and forefinger hold.

4. Compress the breast if it is large, with the finger at the baby's nose to prevent obstruction of breathing.

5. Timing

   a. Feed for 5 minutes per side on the first day.

   b. Feed for 7 to 8 minutes per side on the second day.

   c. Feed for 10 minutes per side on the third day.

   d. Build up to 20 minutes per side.

   e. If the baby falls asleep at 10 minutes, when milk comes in cut back to 5 minutes per side.

   f. If the baby is still hungry, you may go back to the first side for another 5 minutes.

   g. Nurse both breasts at each feeding. Start with the breast you ended with at the last feeding.

   h. At end of the feeding, break the suction by placing your finger in the corner of the baby's mouth.

   i. Air dry the nipples after each feeding and apply Eucerin cream around the areola (brown area) but not on the tip of the nipple. This will keep the nipples from becoming tender.

Breast Massage and Hand Expression

1. Breast massage must be used to bring the milk down to the baby, to relieve fullness, and before pumping or hand expressing to decrease the time spent on collection.

2. To massage: Place one hand under the breast. With the other hand, stroke down toward the nipple, starting from the shoulder. Then stroke under the breast and up. Do this for 1 minute.

3. To hand express: Put the thumb and forefinger on the areola about 1 inch from the nipple. Press back toward the chest wall and squeeze together to compress the milk sinus.

Milk Collection and Storage

1. Milk may be collected and stored when mothers work or are not going to be home for feedings and want the baby to drink from a bottle.

2. Collect milk by hand expression, breast pump, or with milk cups. One ounce at a time may be accumulated, so make sure that enough time is allotted.

3. Collect in a clean container.

4. Chill milk, then freeze. Chilled milk may be poured on top of frozen.

5. Milk may be stored in the refrigerator for 24 to 48 hours only.

6. Glass or plastic bottles or double bagged nursers may be used.

7. Milk can be kept in the back of the freezer for several months.

8. To defrost, run under cold, then warm water, then shake.

9. Discard defrosted milk that the baby does not use.

10. Milk to be transported should be placed in an insulated bag, frozen, or packed with ice.

Breastfeeding Solutions and Problems

1. Soreness
   a. Nipples may become red and cracked or bleeding. The nipple may be sore until it becomes accustomed to baby's sucking, or soreness may be due to poor positioning, removing the baby from the breast improperly, not allowing the nipples to dry, or irritants such as soap, shampoo, rough clothing, plastic liners in bras, or harsh laundry detergents.
   b. Solutions
      1) Rotate the position of the baby when feeding.
      2) Provide short, frequent feedings.
      3) Make sure the baby has the large portion of the nipple in the mouth, not just the tip.
      4) Make sure the baby's mouth is close to the nipple to avoid pulling on the nipple.
      5) Air dry the nipples and use Eucerin cream as necessary.
      6) Nurse on the least sore side first.
      7) Always break suction before removing the baby.
      8) Try saline soaks, ice on the nipples before feeding, a nipple shield or Vitamin E oil if the nipple becomes cracked or bleeds.

2. Fullness or engorgement
   a. Breasts become full on the second or third day postpartum, when the milk comes in. Engorgement is when the milk becomes backed up and the breast and nipples become hard and shiny.

      b. Solutions

        1) Short, frequent feedings help. Do not miss feedings, and nurse on both sides each feeding.

        2) Warm showers, compresses, massage, and expression relieve the fullness.

        3) Make sure the bra is not cutting or binding in any place.

        4) Occasionally expressing or pumping after feeding may relieve fullness.

3. Plugged duct

    a. A plugged duct produces a lump or tenderness in one spot.

    b. Solution

        1) Nurse on the affected breast first.

        2) Direct the baby's chin toward the lump when nursing.

        3) Avoid tight bras, underwire bras, and bunching clothing.

        4) Use massage and heat while nursing to encourage lump drain.

4. Breast infection

    a. Symptoms: flulike feeling, redness, tenderness and fever. The condition may be aggravated by not emptying the breast completely, abrupt weaning, or the mother's fatigue.

    b. Solutions

        1) Heat: warm, moist compresses may help.

        2) Rest will alleviate the mother's fatigue, helping her condition.

        3) Empty the breast completely; when nursing, direct the baby's chin toward a sore spot or lump.

        4) If the client's temperature increases to 100°, call the physician.

Growth Spurts

1. Growth spurts usually come within the first 10 days, at 3 weeks, at 3 months, and at 6 months.

2. The baby may want to nurse more often.

3. Nurse the baby on demand to build up the milk supply.

4. Do not give supplemental feeding, because this may interfere with establishment of an adequate milk supply. The more frequently the breasts are emptied, the more milk is produced.

▧ PARENT EDUCATION PROGRAM: EXPRESSING BREAST MILK

Breast milk may be expressed and collected for later use by hand expression, a hand-operated breast pump, or a semi-automatic battery-operated or electric breast pump. A sterile container, such as sterile plastic bottle bags (Playtex, Gerber, or store brand liners) or a sterilized plastic or glass bottle, should be used to collect the milk. Before collecting milk, wash your hands with soap and water and dry them thoroughly.

Massage each breast in this way. If large-breasted, support the breast with one hand. Beginning at the chest wall, use the other flattened hand to exert gentle pressure on the breast toward the nipple, working around the breast. Work in the areas of greatest milk duct development, under the breast and along the side under the arm. Use the palms of the hands, not the fingers, for firm pressure.

Stimulate the let-down reflex or milk ejection reflex by gently rolling and tugging the nipples between your thumb and forefinger. Dripping of milk from the nipples is one sign that the let-down or milk ejection reflex is working. When you feel that the let-down reflex has begun to work, you can begin expressing breast milk by the chosen method.

Collecting milk may take about 20 minutes. Alternate the breast from which you are expressing milk about four times; when the milk flow slows down on one breast, switch to the other breast. (See Table 4-1.)

A breast pump collection kit should be washed daily in soap and water and rinsed between uses. A dishwasher (which leaves no soap residue) provides an excellent method for cleaning the kit. When collecting milk for a hospitalized infant, the collection kit must the sterilized daily.

PARENT EDUCATION PROGRAM: STORAGE OF HUMAN MILK

Containers

For hospitalized infants, ask your baby's nurse for storage containers. For home use, the following containers and methods are recommended.

1. Clean heavy plastic or glass containers.

2. Disposable bottle liners; double bags are more sturdy.

3. Seal with a lid or twist tie and store upright until frozen.

4. Label the container with the date on which the milk was expressed

Storage

For hospitalized infants, milk should be refrigerated within 1 hour of expressing. In general, use the following guidelines.

1. Milk may be kept at room temperature.

   a. Colostrum: 12 to 24 hours

   b. Mature milk: 6 to 10 hours

TABLE 4-1.
Breast Pumping Schedule

	Right Breast	Left Breast	Right Breast	Left Breast
Day 1	2 min	2 min	2 min	2 min
Day 2	3 min	3 min	3 min	3 min
Day 3	4 min	4 min	4 min	4 min
Day 4	5 min	5 min	5 min	5 min

2. Milk may be refrigerated.

    a. Home use: up to 5 days

    b. Hospitalized infants: up to 48 hours

3. Milk may be frozen.

    a. Home use: 2 weeks in a freezer compartment located inside a refrigerator

    b. Home use: 6 months in a refrigerator/freezer with separate doors (frost free)

    c. Home use: 6 months to 1 year in a deep freeze, 0°F or below

    d. Hospitalized infants: 3 months

Warming Milk

Thaw and/or heat milk by placing the container in warm water. Human milk heats to a comfortable feeding temperature in about 10 minutes.

■ PARENT EDUCATION PROGRAM: HOME PHOTOTHERAPY

1. The unit should be used continuously except when bathing your infant, unless otherwise instructed.

2. A visiting nurse will obtain daily bilirubin blood samples, deliver the samples to a lab, and notify both you and your infant's health care provider of the results.

3. Take your baby's temperature every 8 hours throughout the course of home phototherapy. Because the fiberoptic blanket is not a heat source, temperature instability may signal a problem such as an infection.

4. Monitor the number of wet diapers and record on the flowsheet.

5. Monitor the number and the consistency of bowel movements and record this information on the flowsheet. Your infant may have loose, green-tinged bowel movements as the bilirubin begins to break down.

6. For the bottlefed infant, note and record the amount of formula taken and the frequency of feeding. Feedings should be every 3 hours.

7. For the breastfed infant, note and record the length and frequency of nursing. Feedings should be every 3 hours.

8. Supplement formula or breastfeeding with glucose water unless otherwise instructed.

9. Leave the child on his or her stomach for 1 to 2 hours after eating. Never position the infant on his or her back.

10. The illuminator box should be placed only on a hard, flat surface no more than 4 feet from where the baby will be positioned. Be sure that the air vent in the rear of the unit is not blocked. Use a table or stand next to the baby's bed or the seat where you will be sitting to hold or nurse the baby. Do not put the illuminator next to or on a radiator or heater.

11. Insert the metal collar of the fiberoptic panel completely into the insert of the illuminator. The end of the metal collar of the fiberoptic panel is designed to be even with the end of the insert of the illuminator. Turn the metal collar of the panel clockwise one quarter-turn, to lock it in place.

12. Plug the illuminator box into an electrical outlet. You will need a three-pronged plug (grounded) outlet close by for the electrical cord. A heavy-duty extension cord, such as those used for power tools or appliances, can be used.

13. Insert the panel into a disposable panel cover, ensuring that the light faces the fabric side of the cover, ***not*** the plastic side.

14. Proper placement of the fiberoptic panel will prevent possible skin irritation under the baby's arms. Follow the directions below to assure proper placement:

    a. Place the covered panel around the baby, under his or her arms. Be sure that the fabric side goes against the skin. The lower part of the panel will be on the outside of the baby's diaper. Be sure the diaper is folded down below the baby's navel in front and as far as possible in back so that as much of the skin as possible is exposed to the light.

    b. Using two of the tape tabs provided, fasten the panel in place by affixing the tabs on the plastic side of the cover at the open end, close to where you inserted the fiberoptic panel. ***Do not wrap the baby too tightly.*** A good rule of thumb is to place two fingers between the panel and the baby's skin.

    c. You can now place a T-shirt on the baby, and wrap the child in a blanket or a sleeper.

    d. In larger or more active babies, to prevent possible skin irritation under the baby's arms, tuck a little of the baby's T-shirt, blanket, or sleeper into the top of the panel. Doing this will help cushion the armpit area, preventing skin irritation. You may also use breast shields under the baby's arms.

15. You may now switch on the illuminator and start treatment.

16. You may pick up your baby at any time to hold the child. You can rock, cuddle, or feed the baby. Do not walk around with the baby wrapped in the blanket unit, as you could trip and fall, injuring yourself or the baby. Stay close enough to the illuminator box that it is not pulled off its stand or table.

17. Call your pediatric care provider in the following situations:

    a. If your child is refusing feedings

    b. If there are persistent temperature control problems

    c. If your child has fewer than five wet diapers over a 24-hour period

    d. If there is a pronounced change in your child's level of activity

    e. If your child vomits entire feedings

Box 6-1 is a sample parent information sheet for use in emergencies.

BOX 6-1: PARENT INFORMATION SHEET

Pediatric Provider Phone Number: _______________________________________

Agency Phone Number: ____

TROUBLESHOOTING: If the fiberoptic panel does not light, check all connections. If it still does not light, call the agency office.

■ PARENT EDUCATION PROGRAM: MANAGEMENT OF SEIZURE ACTIVITY

In managing any kind of seizure activity, it is important that you, the parent, remain calm. Explain to others what seizure activity is, particularly those who have or will observe it (siblings, relatives, etc.).

When Your Child Has a Seizure

Keep a record of how often your child has a seizure, noting the times each seizure begins and ends. The most important thing is you can do is protect your child from harm or injury.

If your child has petit mal seizures (gazing into space, daydreaming, or rapid blinking), *seizures* (dreamlike state with meaningless lipsmacking, chewing, grimacing, or repeating words for no reason), or *akinetic seizures* (head drop): There is nothing you can do that has not already been stated here.

If your child has generalized seizures (jerking movements of body, arms, and legs): Ease the child to the floor, couch, or bed and loosen clothing (collars, belts). Remove objects from the area that may cause injury. Do not restrain or interfere with the child; an attempt to limit the jerking movements could cause injury to the child. If possible, turn the child's head to one side so that secretions (saliva) will drain out of the mouth, reducing the possibility of choking. Do not put anything into the child's mouth.

When the seizure is over, your child may want to rest or sleep and may complain of muscle soreness or a headache. Do not offer food or drink until you are sure your child is alert and able to swallow. Reassure your child that he or she is all right.

When to Call the Doctor

1. If seizures are occurring more often and/or lasting longer than usual.

2. If your child seems to pass from one seizure to another without regaining consciousness.

3. If you have any unanswered questions.

Reminders

1. Give your child medication as directed.

2. Do not give your child any medications that contain antihistamines, which can cause an increase in seizure activity.

3. Answer questions honestly.

4. Promote your child's independence. A child with relatively well-controlled seizure activity is able to lead a normal, active life. Provide supervision as necessary.

5. A safety helmet may be needed.

▨ PARENT EDUCATION PROGRAM: INFANT STIMULATION

Infant stimulation is a program of techniques and tools designed to encourage the growth and development of neonates and infants. Infant stimulation is provided to compensate for the limited opportunities that long-term hospitalized infants have or to augment the activities of an average infant. It is a technique that should be based on the four R's of infant stimulation.

1. Rhythm
   All stimulation techniques should be rhythmical, steady, and unforced.

2. Reciprocity
   All infant stimulation should be reciprocal—should involve interaction, "give and take," between the child and the stimulator. The stimulator must be involved.

3. Repetition
   All infant stimulation activities and techniques should involve repetition to promote better learning, to improve neural pathway development, to provide security, and to maintain goals and skills achieved.

4. Reinforcement
   All infant stimulation activities should provide positive and genuine reinforcement of the worth of the infant as an individual. Reinforcement heightens self-esteem and strengthens the bond and attachment between the infant and the stimulator. The infant and stimulator must approach this as fun time.

Infant stimulation has a profound effect upon the mental, physical, and emotional development of each infant. It enhances the mental development of the infant by stimulating curiosity, cultivating a longer attention span, and promoting more age-appropriate play skills. Infant stimulation affects the physical growth of the infant by promoting better muscle coordination and better muscle control, and infants tend to gain weight faster. Emotionally, infants tend to establish strong attachments, trust that their needs will be met, have a sense of control over their environment, smile sooner and more frequently, are content, and have a secure self-image.

Parents should be encouraged to perform infant stimulation activities. Infant stimulation provided in the home by a consistent caretaker is important to the recently hospitalized infant because these infants receive less individual handling and therefore less stimulation. They are separated from their parents for longer time frames, which interferes with the bonding process and lessens the quality of parent–child interaction. They are often deprived of normal newborn experiences.

The infant stimulation program should be based upon the child's present level of functioning and upon the child's needs along the developmental continuum. Often, a child will be functioning well in the areas of cognition, language, or social/emotional development, yet due to confinement the child's motor skills will be delayed. Therefore, each child's program should be tailored to meet his or her individual needs; it should be based upon the child's developmental age and should provide for activity development in each skill area. Activities selected should encourage age-appropriate play skills while taking into consideration the child's medical situation, developmental age, and capabilities. Infants suspected of delays in any of these areas should be referred to the local early intervention program for evaluation.

Below is a list of suggested play activities and toys for the infant, according to age.

1. 1 month: Provide mobiles, rattles, black-and-white objects, and bright simple pictures lining the crib. The baby enjoys leg/arm cycling and smiles at faces.

2. 2 months: The baby enjoys listening to a variety of sounds, therefore talk and sing to him or her often. Lay the baby on his or her stomach and lay on your stomach with your head facing the baby's. Try to get the baby to hold up his or her head and make eye contact. The baby will also respond to voices.

3. 3 months: Peek-a-boo games encourage discovery. Provide soft, safe, furry cuddle toys. Mount a mirror for the baby.

4. 4 months: Allow some time for the baby to play alone. Encourage movement and rolling. The baby will also react to sounds.

5. 5 months: Provide durable, washable toys with handles. Begin "Pat-a-cake" songs and "So Big" games with gestures. Encourage rocking, wriggling, and rolling by placing objects at arm's length away; this will also encourage the baby to reach out and grab.

6. 6 months: Play "Where's baby?" Play knee games and tummy tickles. The baby will like to laugh and squeal.

7. 7 months: Play hold the baby's hands and encourage standing/walking motion.

8. 8 months: Imitate the baby. Chase the baby. Provide pull toys, stacking blocks, and building blocks.

9. 9 months: The baby will enjoy toys to be picked up with the fingers, push/pull toys, and musical toys.

10. 10 months: Baby books, baby blocks, and children's music are appropriate.

11. 11 months: Riding toys pushed by feet and pop-up toys are suitable.

12. 12 months: Push/pull toys, baby books, children's music, and short videos are appropriate.

PARENT EDUCATION PROGRAM: EMERGENCY CARE GUIDE

Important Numbers

Emergency Medical Services: _______________________________

Poison Control Center: _______________________________

Family Doctor: _______________________________

Bites and Stings

Call 911 (or the local emergency number) immediately if a bite wound is bleeding severely. Proceed as for *Bleeding*, described below. Also do this if the wound is deep or from an unknown animal. If the wound is not bleeding profusely, wash the area with mild soap and running water while you wait for help to arrive, but do not use ointments or creams. If any tissue has been bitten off, wrap it in a clean, wet cloth, place it in a plastic bag, and bring it with you to the hospital. If the child has been stung, call 911 (or the local emergency number) if he or she shows signs of a severe allergic reaction such as shock, wheezing, or spreading rash or welts. This can be life-threatening!!!

Bleeding

Try to control the bleeding by applying direct pressure to the wound or cut with a clean cloth. Elevate the wounded area unless you suspect a broken bone. Call 911 (or the local emergency number) if the bleeding cannot be controlled or if there is a puncture wound caused by a large or embedded object. If the wound seems deep or gaping and you suspect the child needs stitches, go to the hospital emergency room.

Broken Bones and Head/Spine Injuries

In situations such as car accidents, falls greater than the child's height, or significant trauma to the head or spine, assume there is a head or spine injury. Call 911 (or the local emergency number) immediately. Do not move the child; keep him or her still. Control any bleeding (see *Bleeding*, above). For broken bones, immobilize the injured part with a splint—only if you have been properly trained in the technique—and call 911 (or the local emergency number).

Burns

1. If burns are on the child's face, hands, feet, or genitals, or if they are white, blistered, or charred, or larger than the size of the child's hand, call 911 (or the local emergency number). While waiting for paramedics to arrive, cover the burns with a clean, cool, wet towel or sheet, or flush with cool water. For open wounds, use a dry towel.

2. For chemical burns, flush the area with running water until help arrives. Remove any of the child's clothing or jewelry saturated with the chemical as soon as possible.

3. For electrical burns or shock, do not touch the child until you have separated him or her from the power source by turning off the electricity. Check breathing and pulse, then call 911 (or the local emergency number).

4. For minor burns, flush the area with cool water and call the family doctor for follow-up care. Never use ointments, creams, or butter without consulting a physician.

Dental Emergencies

Carefully remove any tooth fragments from the mouth. Do not clean the tooth or remove any tissue attached to it; submerge it in a glass of milk (or water if milk is not available) and take both the child and the tooth to the dentist immediately.

Drowning

Begin cardiopulmonary resuscitation as needed on an unconscious child. If the child's pulse has stopped, have someone call 911 (or the local emergency number) while you begin CPR (see *No Pulse* below).

Poisoning

If the child has any extreme symptoms—such as unconsciousness, breathing difficulties, or seizures—call 911 (or the local emergency number). Otherwise, call the area Poison Control Center, specifying the substance involved, how much was ingested, and the child's age, weight, and condition. Have syrup of ipecac on hand, but do not induce vomiting unless instructed to do so. If you are told to go to a hospital, take the poisonous substance container along.

Any First-Aid Situation (except spine injuries)

After you have given specific care, lay the child on his or her back, elevate the legs slightly, and keep his or her body at a comfortable temperature until help arrives.

Choking

1. Infants up to 12 months

   a. If the baby is coughing forcefully, do not interfere or you may make the situation worse; allow the obstruction to clear itself.

   b. If the infant cannot cough, breathe, or cry:

      1) Stand or sit with him face down along your forearm, resting your arm on your thigh so that the baby's head is lower than his chest; cup his jaw with your hand. With the heel of your other hand, give four quick, firm blows to his back between the shoulder blades.

      2) If this does not dislodge the item, turn the baby onto his back, keeping his head lowered. Give four chest thrusts, with two fingers placed on the breastbone one finger's-width below the imaginary line connecting the nipples. Compress the breastbone $1/2$ to 1 inch with each thrust.

      3) Repeat the combination of back blows and chest thrusts until the object comes out or until the infant becomes unconscious In either case, have the baby checked later for internal injuries.

   c. If the infant loses consciousness, roll the infant onto his or her back; avoid twisting the body and neck. Open the airway by tilting the head back gently. Push down on the forehead until the chin points up and the mouth drops open.

2. Children 12 months and older

   a. If the child is coughing forcefully, talking, or breathing, don't do anything; allow the obstruction to clear itself.

   b. For a conscious child who cannot breathe at all, perform the Heimlich maneuver. Bring your arms around the child from behind. Make a fist, and place the thumb side against the middle of the abdomen just above the navel. Grab your fist with your other hand and press in with quick, upward thrusts. Repeat until the object comes out or the child becomes unconscious.

   c. If the child loses consciousness:

     1) Roll the child onto his or her back; avoid twisting the neck and back. Open the airway by tilting the head back gently. Push down on the forehead while lifting the chin. Look, listen, and feel breathing for 3 to 5 seconds. If the child shows no sign of breathing, pinch the nose shut and cover the mouth with yours. Blow in two puffs of air, taking a breath in between. Watch the chest as you do this; if it does not rise, re-tilt the head and do it again.

     2) If the chest still does not rise, administer blows and thrusts as for *Choking*, above. Then do a foreign-object check. Open the mouth, holding the tongue down with your thumb. If you can see an object (and only if you can see one), remove it by sweeping your little finger with a hook action along the base of the tongue. Repeat the cycle of head-tilt/chin-lift, two breaths, blows and thrusts, and object check until breaths go in.

     3) If breaths do go in, check for a pulse for 5 to 10 seconds with two fingers placed on the inside of the child's upper arm midway between the elbow and the armpit. If there is a pulse, but still no breathing, continue breathing into the mouth and nose once every 3 seconds. If you cannot detect a pulse within 10 seconds, start CPR (see *No Pulse*, below).

No Pulse

1. If the infant is not breathing and has no pulse, give CPR. Place two fingers on the breastbone, one finger's-width below the nipple line. Push the chest downward $1/2$ to 1 inch and release, five times in quick succession (within 3 seconds). Then give one breath (as in *Choking*, item 2.c.1, above). Continue CPR for 1 minute, then recheck the pulse. If there is no pulse, give one rescue breath and continue CPR until the pulse resumes or help arrives.

2. When breaths do go in, check for a pulse on the side of the neck. If there is a pulse but still no breathing, continue breathing into the mouth once every 4 seconds. If you cannot detect a pulse within 10 seconds, start CPR.

Unconsciousness and Choking

Give 6 to 10 quick upward thrusts with the heel of your hand placed just above the navel. Then open the mouth, holding the tongue down with your thumb; if you can see a foreign object, remove it by sweeping your little finger with a hook action along the base of the tongue. Repeat the cycle of head-tilt/chin-lift, two breaths, blows and thrusts, and object check until breaths go in(as in *Choking*, item 2.c.1, above).

PARENT EDUCATION PROGRAM: BASIC HOME SAFETY

Fire Safety (to eliminate fire hazards)

1. The furnace and water heater should be checked at least once a year to ensure safety.

2. Wood stoves or portable heaters should be installed properly, and chimneys should be cleaned and inspected once a year.

3. Flammable liquids should be stored outside, away from any heat source, and disposed of properly.

4. Electrical appliances should be used safely and checked periodically.

5. Matches, cigarettes, and smoking materials should be disposed of safely in an ashtray or fire-resistant container.

6. The kitchen stove should be kept free of grease. No loose-fitting clothes should be worn when cooking. Pot handles should be turned away from the front of the stove and potholders always should be used.

7. Oxygen should be used away from open flames and heat. Do not place concentrator near a heat source. Tubing should not come in contact with stoves, space heaters, or baseboard heating coils. Do not use electrical devices, such as electric razors, while using oxygen. Post "NO SMOKING" signs. Clean up any oil or grease before using oxygen (as it may combine with oxygen and spontaneously ignite).

8. Develop a fire safety plan.
   a. Standard fire regulations recommend one smoke detector on every level of the home.
   b. Develop an evacuation plan for use in case of fire. Note which family members will require assistance because of age, illness, or disability.
   c. Establish clear pathways to all exits. Do not block exits with furniture or boxes.
   d. Have keys stored near doors locked with deadbolts.
   e. Do not leave cooking unattended for long periods of time.
   f. Chimneys should be inspected annually to avoid dangerous buildup of creosote.
   g. Kerosene heaters, wood stoves, and fireplaces should not be left unattended while in use. Never use a gas stove for space heating.
   h. Have a fire extinguisher in an easily accessible place (e.g., kitchen).

Electrical Safety

1. Cords must not be placed beneath furniture or rugs.

2. Replace frayed cords.

3. Do not overload extension cords. Check rating labels on cords and appliances.

4. Multiple outlet adapters should not be used on electrical outlets.

5. Cover unused outlets, and teach young children not to touch plugs, cords, or outlets.

6. Never replace a fuse with a penny or a higher amp fuse. Use correctly sized fuses at all times.

7. Never turn on an appliance or plug one in while standing in water or if your hands are wet.

8. Call a professional electrician if you suspect an electrical problem. Blown fuses or dimmed lights may indicate a wiring problem.

9. Make sure the electrical system is sufficient when using medical equipment such as ventilators and oxygen concentrators. Check with the medical supplier or an electrician.

10. Use three-pronged adapters when required.

11. When ambulating with a pump, IV pole, electrical cord, or IV tubing, carefully position the equipment between you and the outlet, to avoid falls or electrical accidents.

Environmental Safety

1. Loose rugs, runners, and mats should be secured to the floor with double-sided tape or rubber matting.

2. Carpet edges should be tacked down.

3. Torn, worn, frayed carpeting should be repaired, replaced, or removed.

4. Cupboards should be organized so that frequently used items are on lower shelves.

5. A sturdy stepstool should be used to reach items on high shelves.

6. Heavy items should be stored flat on lower levels of the closet to avoid falls and injury.

7. Stairs, hallways, and passageways between rooms should be well lit and free of clutter.

8. Stairs should have sturdy, well-secured handrails on both sides. Install gates, if needed, to protect children from falls.

9. Avoid using stairs while wearing only socks or smooth-soled shoes.

10. Furniture should be arranged to allow free movement in heavy traffic areas.

11. Hazardous tools and firearms should be kept locked up. Unplug appliances and tools when not in use.

12. Cleaning fluids, polishes, bleaches, detergents, and all poisons should be stored separately and clearly marked. Proper ventilation should be available when cleaning fluids are being used.

13. Spills should be cleaned up promptly.

14. Old newspapers and cleaning cloths should not be stockpiled.

15. Insects, rodents, and bad odors should be controlled.

16. Place at least one phone in a position that is accessible in the event that an accident renders a person unable to stand. Emergency numbers should be posted near the phone, including ambulance, doctor, fire, police, and poison control.

17. Entrance ways should be clear of leaves, snow, and ice.

Bathroom Safety

1. Tubs and showers should have a textured surface or nonskid mats or strips to prevent falls.

2. Grab-bars to assist transfers should be installed in tub, showers, and toilet areas when applicable.

3. Check the water temperature with your hand before entering the tub or shower. The water temperature setting may need to be lowered.

4. A night light should be used in the bathroom if possible.

5. A bell, buzzer, or appropriate noisemaker should be placed in the bathroom for emergency use.

6. Ground fault outlets should be installed.

7. Electrical appliances should be used away from water.

8. The door lock should be a type that can be opened from the outside in an emergency.

9. Never leave a child alone in the bathtub. ***A child can drown in a few inches of water!!!***

10. If possible, locate a bathroom on the first floor.

Bibliography

Alaska Department of Health and Social Services: *Alaska Maternal and Child Health Manual for Public Health Nursing*. Alaska Department of Health and Social Services, Division of Public Health, Section of Nursing, Anchorage, Alaska; June 1994.

American Diabetes Association: *Medical Management of Pregnancy Complicated by Diabetes*. American Diabetes Association, Alexandria, Virginia; 1993.

Arkin, Elaine Bratic, and Judith E. Funkhouser: *Communicating About Alcohol and Other Drugs: Strategies for Reaching Populations at Risk*. U.S. Department of Public Health and Human Services, Rockville, Maryland; 1990.

Association of Maternal and Child Health Programs: *Caring for Mothers and Children. A Report of a Survey of FY 1987 State MCH Program Activities*. Association of Maternal and Child Health Programs, Washington, D.C.; March 1989.

Association of Maternal and Child Health Programs: *Toward the Future of Title V! A Report on Site Visits to Ten State Programs*. Association of Maternal and Child Health Programs, Washington, D.C.; November 1991.

Association of Maternal and Child Health Programs: *Meeting Needs, Building Capacities. State Perspectives on Graduate Training and Continuing Education Needs of Title V Programs*. Association of Maternal and Child Health Programs, Washington, D.C.; October 1992.

Association of Women's Health, Obstetric, and Neonatal Nurses: *Practice Resource: Preparation for Technology-Dependent Infants*. Association of Women's Health, Obstetric, and Neonatal Nurses, McLean VA; January 1993.

Bass, Alison: Few support services are available once ill children go home. *Boston Sunday Globe*, November 27, 1988.

Betz, Cecily Lynn, et al.: Altered digestive function. *Family Centered Nursing Care of Infants*, 35:1478–1480; 1994.

Block, Carol, et al.: *Home Care for High-Risk Infants, The First Year. Caring*, pp. 11–17. National Association for Home Care, Washington, D.C.; May 1989.

Boland, Mary G., and Lynn Czarniecki: Starting life with HIV, *RN*, pp. 54–58; January 1991.

Bradley, Robert, and Bettye Caldwell: Using the HOME inventory to assess the family environment. *Pediatric Nursing*, 14(2):97–102; March–April 1988.

Briggs, Nancy: Hospitals & home care: Inseparable in the '80's. *Pediatric Nursing*, 12(5):384–385; September–October 1986.

Briggs, Nancy, Connie Lierman, Julie Hazelton, Richard Wolff, Kinny Pasquera, and Elizabeth Wilson: Multidisciplinary treatment of feeding disorders in the home. *Pediatric Nursing*, 13(4):266–271; July–August 1987.

Britton, John R., and Helen Britton: Efficacy of early newborn discharge in a middle-class population. *MDC*, 138:1041–1045; November 1984.

Britton, John R., Helen Britton, and Susan Beebe: Early discharge of the term newborn: A continued dilemma. *Pediatrics*, 94(3):291–295; September 1994.

Brown, Sarah S., ed.: *Prenatal Care. Reaching Mothers. Reaching Infants*. National Academy Press, Washington, D.C.; 1988.

Boyer, D.: Prediction of postpartum depression. *NAACOG Clinical Issues in Perinatal and Women's Health Nursing*, 1(3):267–278; 1990.

Casey, Robert P.: *Investing in Our Children and Families, 1993–94 Budget Initiatives*. Executive Office, Harrisburg, Pennsylvania; 1993.

Casey, Robert P.: *Managed Competition: A Health Care System for Pennsylvania*. Report of the Pennsylvania Economic Development Partnership Health Care Committee to The Pennsylvania Economic Development Partnership. Executive Office, Harrisburg, Pennsylvania; November 1992.

Child Health Foundation: Diarrhea kills over 300 U.S. children annually. *NEWS, Child Health Foundation Newsletter*, Columbia, Maryland; June 2, 1996.

Children's Hospital of Los Angeles: *Informational Guidelines for Parents*. Children's Hospital of Los Angeles, Nutrition Support Program, Los Angeles; 1990.

Children's Hospital of Philadelphia: *Informational Guidelines for Parents*. Children's Hospital of Philadelphia, Nutrition Support Program, Philadelphia; 1991.

Commonwealth of Pennsylvania, Department of Health: *Maternal and Child Health Services*. Draft Block Grant Application, Federal Fiscal Year 1993. Pennsylvania Department of Health, Harrisburg, Pennsylvania; 1993.

Commonwealth of Pennsylvania, Department of Health: *Guide to Health Data for Pennsylvania*. State Health Data Center, Harrisburg, Pennsylvania; June 1996.

Commonwealth of Pennsylvania, Department of Public Welfare: *Pennsylvania Medical Assistance Program Eligibility Verification System Manual*. Publication 261. Pennsylvania Department of Public Welfare, Harrisburg, Pennsylvania; April 1993.

Commonwealth of Pennsylvania, Department of Public Welfare: Statistics provided by outpatient staff. Pennsylvania Department of Public Welfare, Harrisburg, Pennsylvania; May 13, 1993.

Commonwealth of Pennsylvania, Department of Public Welfare: *Overview, The Family Care Network*. Pennsylvania Department of Public Welfare, Harrisburg, Pennsylvania; 1994.

Cook, Paddy, Robert Petersen, and Dorothy Moore: *Alcohol, Tobacco, and Other Drugs May Harm the Newborn*. United States Department of Health and Human Services, Rockville, Maryland; 1990.

Cornelius, Llewellyn B.: Barriers to medical care for white, black, and Hispanic American children. *Journal of the National Medical Association*, 85(4):281–288; 1993.

Corporation for Public Broadcasting: *Miracle of Life*. Video production airing on public broadcasting series NOVA. Corporation for Public Broadcasting, Films for Humanities and Sciences, Monmouth Junction, New Jersey; 1983.

Craven, Ruth F.: *Fundamentals of Nursing*, 2nd edition. Lippincott–Raven Publishers, Philadelphia; 1996.

Cunningham, Gary, and Marshall Lindheimer: Hypertension in pregnancy. *New England Journal of Medicine*, 326(14):927–931; 1992.

Davis, Matthew, ed.: *Health Care Reform Update*, 1(8). National Association for Home Care; Washington, D.C.; May 12, 1993.

Dingell, John D., and Committee of Conference: *Conference Report, ADAMNA Reorganization Act. Title V. Home Visiting Services for At-Risk Families*. 102nd Congress, 2nd Session, House of Representatives, Report 102-546. U.S. House of Representatives, Washington, D.C.; 1994.

Donar, Mary: Community care: Pediatric home mechanical ventilation. *Holistic Nursing Practice*, 2(2):68–80; 1988.

Falkner, F., ed.: *Prevention of Infant Mortality and Morbidity. Child Health and Development*, Volume 4. Karger, Basel, Switzerland; 1985.

Farber, Anne E.: *Survey of Home Visiting Programs for Children and Families in Pennsylvania, Executive Summary*. University of Pittsburgh, University Center for Social and Urban Reseach, Office of Child Development, Pittsburgh, Pennsylvania; 1996.

Fitzgerald, Susan: 1 in 6 New mothers used cocaine, study finds. *Philadelphia Inquirer*; April 8, 1989.

Fitzgerald, Susan: How three nations shape birth. *Philadelphia Inquirer, Suburban Edition*; April 27, 1993.

Friesen, Barbara J., Joanne Griesbach, Judith Jacobs, Judith Katz-Leavy, and Dennis Olson: Improving services for families. *Children Today*, pp. 18–22; July–August 1988.

Federal Register: Medicare regulations. *Federal Register: Rules and Regulations*, 54(153); August 14, 1989.

Fleming, Barbara W.: Assessing and promoting positive parenting in adolescent mothers. *MCN*, 18:32–37; January–February 1993.

Grabert, B., C. Wardell, and S. Harburg: Home phototherapy. *Clinical Pediatrics*, 25:291–294; 1986.

Harrison, H., and A. Kositsky: *The Premature Baby Book*. St. Martin's Press, New York; 1983.

Henrikson, Mary, Ginna Wall, Dona Lethbridge, and Vicki McClurg: Nursing diagnosis and obstetric, gynecologic, and neonatal nursing: Breastfeeding as an example. *JOGN Thoughts and Opinions*, 21(6); November–December 1992.

Herman, Robin: France wants me to have this baby. *Washington Post*; May 1, 1990.

Hoerlin, Bettina Yaffe: *Targeting for the Future: Health Care in the Philadelphia Region*. Report to The Pew Charitable Trusts, Philadelphia, Pennsylvania; January 1989.

Howard, Tracy: *Kids Ending Hunger. What Can We Do?* Andrews and McMeel, A Universal Press Syndicate Co., Kansas City, Missouri; 1992.

Hyde-Robertson, Barbara L.: The necessity for maternal–infant perinatal home care. *Caring*, pp. 26–31. National Association for Home Care, Washington, D.C.; December 1992.

Infante-Rivard, Claire, Gisele Filion, Mona Baumgarten, Madeleine Bourassa, Johanne Labelle, and Monique Messier: A public health home intervention among families of low socioeconomic status. *CHC*, 18(2):102; Spring 1989.

Institute of Medicine: *Nutrition During Pregnancy and Lactation*. National Academy Press, Washington, D.C.; 1990.

Johns Hopkins Oral Rehydration Project: *Outpatient Oral Rehydration Therapy Protocol*. Johns Hopkins Oral Rehydration Project, Baltimore, Maryland; 1991.

Johnson, S., and D. Kraut: *Pregnancy and Bedrest: A Guide for the Pregnant Woman and Her Family*. St. Martin's Press, New York; 1990.

Langevin, Jeanne: Using home health aids in a high-risk infant program. *Caring,* pp. 40–43. National Association for Home Care, Washington, D.C.; June 1988.

Marecki, Marsha: Postpartum followup goals and assessment. *JOGN*, pp. 214–218; August 1979.

Marks, Margaret G.: *Introductory Pediatric Nursing*, 4th edition. Lippincott–Raven Publishers, Philadelphia; 1994.

McAnarney, Elizabeth R.: Experience with an adolescent health care program. *Public Health Reports*, 90(5):412–416; September–October 1975.

McAnarney, Elizabeth R.: Development of an adolescent maternity project in Rochester, New York. *Public Health Reports*, 92(2):154–159; March–April 1977.

NAACOG: *Criteria Established for Identifying At-Risk Infants*, 14(10). NAACOG, Washington, D.C.; October 1987.

NAACOG: *OGN Nursing Practice Resource: Neonatal Skin Care*. NAACOG, Washington, D.C.; 1992.

National Center for Education in Maternal and Child Health: *Reaching Out: A Directory of National Organizations Related to Maternal and Child Health*. National Center for Education in Maternal and Child Health, Washington, D.C.; March 1989.

National Commission to Prevent Infant Mortality: *One Stop Shopping: A Road to Healthy Mothers and Children*. National Commission to Prevent Infant Mortality: Washington, D.C., April 1991.

Nettina, Sandra M.: *Lippincott Manual of Nursing Practice*, 6th edition. Lippincott–Raven Publishers, Philadelphia; 1996.

North Carolina Department of Health: *MCH Manual*. Department of Public Health, Durham, North Carolina; 1992.

Nuttal, P.: Maternal responses to home apnea monitoring of infants. *Nursing Research*, 37:354–357; 1988.

Oehler, Jerri N., et al.: How to target infants at highest risk for developmental delay. *Maternal–Child Nursing*, 18:20–23; January–February 1993.

Olds, D.: The prenatal/infancy project: A strategy for responding to the needs of high risk mothers and their children. *Prevention in Human Services*, 7(1):59–87; 1989.

Olds, D., C. Henderson, R. Tatlebaum, and R. Chamberlin: Improving the delivery of prenatal care and outcomes of pregnancy: A randomized trial of nurse home visitation. *Pediatrics*, 77(1):16–28; January 1986.

Olds, D., and H. Kitzman: Can home visitation improve the health of women and children at environmental risk? *Pediatrics*, 1(1):108–116; July 1990.

Pennsylvania Department of Health: *Block Grant, Commonwealth of Pennsylvania Preventive and Primary Care Services for Pregnant Women, Mothers, and Infants up to Age 1, Component A*, p. 64. Pennsylvania Department of Health, Division of Maternal Child Health, Harrisburg, Pennsylvania.

Pennsylvania Department of Health: *Vital Statistics 1990*. Pennsylvania Department of Health, State Health Data Center, Harrisburg, Pennsylvania; 1992.

Pennsylvania Healthy Mothers, Healthy Babies Coalition: *Pennsylvania Healthy Mothers, Healthy Babies Coalition* Pennsylvania Healthy Mothers, Healthy Babies Coalition, Bryn Mawr, Pennsylvania; 1992.

Pennsylvania Partnerships for Children: *Our Children, Our Future.* Breakfast on Children's Health Issues. Pennsylvania Partnerships for Children, Harrisburg, Pennsylvania; October 9, 1991.

Pennsylvania Partnerships for Children: *Kids Count.* State Grant Proposal for Pennsylvania. Pennsylvania Partnerships for Children, Harrisburg, Pennsylvania; August 13, 1992.

Perrin, James M.: Chronically ill children, in America, the case for home care. *Journal for Physicians in Home Care*; Spring 1987.

Philadelphia Department of Public Health: *Selected Resident Birth and Death Data by Health District, by Census Tract and by Neighborhood, 1983–1993.* Department of Public Health, Philadelphia, 1994.

Reece, S.: Social support and the early maternal experience for primiparas over 35. *Maternal–Child Nursing Journal*, 3:91–98; July–September 1993.

Reeder, S., L. Martin, and D. Koniak-Griffin: *Maternity Nursing, Family Newborn and Women's Health Care*, 18th edition. Lippincott–Raven Publishers, Philadelphia; 1997.

Richmond, Frederick, Martha Wade Steketee, et al.: *The State of the Child: A Profile of Pennsylvania's Children.* Waldman Graphics, Philadelphia; 1993.

Roberts, Joyce: Current perspectives in preeclampsia. *Journal of Nurse Midwifery*, 39(2):70–90; 1994.

Rogatz, Peter: Perspective on home care. *Public Health Nursing*, 4(1):7–8; March 1987.

Rosen, C., D. Glaze, and J. Frost: Home monitor followup of persistent apnea and bradycardia in preterm infants. *American Journal of Diseases in Children*, 140:547–550; 1986.

Shelton, Terri I., Elizabeth Jeppson, and Beverly Johnson: *Family Centered Care for Children with Special Health Care Needs*, 2nd edition. Association for the Care of Children's Health, U.S. Public Health Service, Division of Maternal Child Health, Rockville, Maryland; 1987.

Sills, Joanne: Infant deaths soar in areas. *Philadelphia Daily News*; July 8, 1992.

Sirkka, L.: Health promotion in child and family health care: The role of the Finnish public health nurses. *Public Health Nursing*, 11(1):32–37; February 1994.

Smith, Judy: The dangers of prenatal cocaine use. *Maternal–Child Nursing*, 13:174–179; May–June 1992.

South Carolina Department of Health and Environmental Control: *Comprehensive Risk Screening for Patient Referrals.* South Carolina Department of Health and Environmental Control, Maternal Health, Columbia, South Carolina; October 1992.

Stanwick, Richard S., Michael E. K. Moffat, Yvonne Robitaille, Aline Edmond, and Caroline Dok: An evaluation of the routine postnatal public health nurse home visit. *Canadian Journal of Public Health*, 73:200–205; May–June 1982.

Starn, J.: Community health nursing visits for at risk women and infants. *Journal of Community Health Nursing*, 9(2):103–110; 1992.

Streeter, N. S.: Discharge planning home care. *Journal of Perinatal and Neonatal Nursing* 5(1); 1991.

Sullivan, Joan, et al.: Can we help the substance abusing mother and infant? *Maternal–Child Nursing*, 18:153–157; May–June 1993.

United Way of Pennsylvania: *Report of the Success-By-Six Coalition: Helping All Children Succeed for Life.* United Way of Pennsylvania, Harrisburg, Pennsylvania; June 1992.

U.S.D.L., Occupational Safety and Health, Office of Health Compliance Assistance: *OSHA Instruction CPL 2-2, 44A*, p. 4. U.S. Department of Labor Occupational Safety and Health, Office of Health Compliance Assistance, Washington, D.C.; August 15, 1988.

U.S.D.P.H., Agency for Health Care Policy and Research: *The 50 Most Frequent Diagnosis-Related Groups (DRO's), Diagnoses, and Procedures: Statistics by Hospital Size and Location.* Hospital Studies Program Research Note 13. U.S. Department of Public Health, Agency for Health Care Policy and Research, Rockville, Maryland; September 1990.

U.S.D.P.H., Agency for Health Care Policy and Research: *Research Activities: Contracts Awarded for Low Birthweight, Health Care for Women, Barriers to Quality Care Persist.* Publication No. 158. U.S. Department of Public Health, Agency for Health Care Policy and Research, Rockville, Maryland; November 1992.

U.S.D.P.H., Agency for Health Care Policy and Research: *Research Activities: Number of Uninsured Children on the Rise, Less than 15 Percent of America's Health Care Dollar Spent on Children.* Publication No. 162. U.S. Department of Public Health, Agency for Health Care Policy and Research, Rockville, Maryland; March 1993.

U.S.D.P.H., Agency for Health Care Policy and Research: *Research Activities: Women Planning Pregnancy Often Switch to HMO's*. Publication No. 163. U.S. Department of Public Health, Agency for Health Care Policy and Research, Rockville, Maryland; April 1993.

U.S.D.P.H., Agency for Health Care Policy and Research: *Research Activities: Uninsured Patients More Likely to Die Prematurely*. Publication No. 169. U.S. Department of Public Health, Agency for Health Care Policy and Research, Rockville, Maryland; October 1993.

U.S.D.P.H., Agency for Health Care Policy and Research: *Research Activities: Financially Troubled Hospitals Face Difficult Choices, Outlook Poor for Very Young Babies with AIDS, Teen Health Programs Often Deficient in On Site Services*. Publication No. 170. U.S. Department of Public Health, Agency for Health Care Policy and Research, Rockville, Maryland; November 1993.

U.S.D.P.H.H.S.: *Caring for Our Future: The Content of Prenatal Care*. U.S. Department of Public Health and Human Services, Washington, D.C.; 1989.

U.S.P.H.S.: *Back to Sleep: Reducing the Risk of Sudden Infant Death Syndrome—What You Can Do*. The American Academy of Pediatrics, SIDS Alliance,, and the Association of SIDS Program Professionals. U.S. Public Health Service, Washington, D.C.

Vrazo, Fawn: Pregnant doctors in distress. *Philadeinhia Inquirer*; February 17, 1990.

Vrazo, Fawn: Lying in is now out for many new mothers. *Philadelphia Inquirer*; August 17, 1990.

Vrazo, Fawn: Lying in is out as insurers cut post-childbirth coverage. *Philadelphia Inquirer*; August 7, 1993.

Wasik, B., D. Bryant, and C. Lyons: *Home Visiting: Procedures for Helping Families*. Sage Publications, Newbury Park, California; 1990.

Weston, Donna R., Barbara Ivins, Barry Zuckerman, Coryl Jones, and Richard Lopez: *Drug Exposed Babies: Research and Clinical Issues*. National Center for Clinical Infant Programs, Washington, D.C.; June 1989.

Williams, Lenore, and Mary Cooper: Nurse managed postpartum home care. *JOGN Principles and Practice*, pp. 25–31; January–February 1993.

Wisconsin Association for Perinatal Care: *Early Discharge—Short Term Length of Stay*. Wisconsin Association for Perinatal Care; June 1993.

Yariover, Mark J., Deloras Jones, and Michael D. Miller: Perinatal care of low risk mothers and infants. *New England Journal of Medicine*, 294(13):702–705; March 25, 1976.

Young, L., D. Creighton, and R. Sauve: The needs of families of infants discharged home with continous oxygen therapy. *Journal of Obstetric, Gynecolgic, and Neonatal Nursing*, 17:187–193; 1987.

Zuravin, Susan J.: *Child Maltreatment and Teenage First Births: A Relationship Mediated by Chronic Sociodemographic Stress?* American Orthopsychiatric Association, Washington, D.C.; January 1988.

Additional Resources

Free or low-cost educational material can be obtained from the following additional health information resources.

U.S. Department of Health and Human Services
Public Health Service Office of Disease Prevention and Health Promotion
ONHIC, P.O. Box 1133
Washington, DC 20013-1133
(800) 336-4797
Request the *Health Information Resources Catalogue*

Maternal Child Health Bureau
March of Dimes Birth Defects Foundation
National Center for Education in Maternal Child Health
Write to: National Maternal Child Health Clearing House
      8201 Greensboro Drive, Suite 600
      McLean, VA 22102
(703) 821-8955, ext. 254 or 265
Request *Prenatal Care, A Resource Guide*

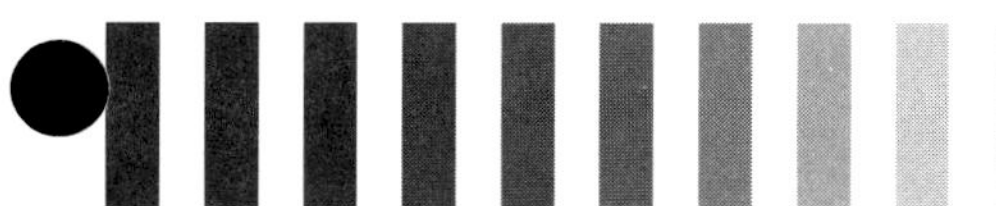

The appendices of this manual contain additional information that the provider will find helpful in creating a well-organized High-Risk Newborn Home Program. Section 1 contains clinical records designed for a High-Risk Newborn Home Care visiting program that also seeks Medicare certification or accreditation through JCAHO or NLN. Included is a copy of the standard Plan of Care developed for use by the Health Care Financing Administration (HCFA; *Appendix A)*. This document records the physician orders for home care services and should be completed by the nurse. Also included are clinical records to be used by the nurse in developing a comprehensive plan of nursing care, but which would also be of use to professionals in other disciplines such as physical therapy and social work. Included in addition to the HCFA form are the following.

1. **Home Health Client Rights and Consent Forms:** Organizations will want to modify this form to assure that clients have the hotline phone number to their individual state surveyor office. For Medicare-certified agencies, allowing clients access to this number is a federal requirement. *(See Appendices B–D.)*
2. **Initial Evaluation Form:** This is to be completed by the nurse as part of the medical assessment for newborns admitted to home care after the first universal assessment. These are newborns who will receive visits according to the Plan of Care outlined on the enclosed HCFA form. *(See Appendix E.)*
3. **Current Medication profile:** This is to be completed by the nurse at the first visit and updated at each subsequent visit. The nurse should always review side effects and contraindications in addition to always verifying the medicaton orders with the prescriptions obtained from the pharmacy. The nurse should never assume that the parents are calculating dosages correctly, and should observe them at least once as they perform these procedures. Although aides do not administer medications, they should be oriented to this in order to be more familiar with the client's needs. *(See Appendix F.)*
4. **Nursing Plan of Care and Progress Record:** This is to be used by the nurse for subsequent home visits. *(See Appendix G.)*
5. **Nursing Progress Notes:** This is for use by nurses and aides. Home health aides should summarize care each visit or shift. *(See Appendix H.)*
6. **Pediatric Intake and Output:** A clinical record tool the nurse may find helpful to have the client's family and the aide maintain. It should be reviewed by the nurse on each visit. *(See Appendix I.)*
7. **Home Needs Assessment Form:** This tool is not a required, but is helpful in obtaining additional information about the homes of children whose care requires technological support. Prior to hospital discharge, questions such as "Does the child's home have adequate electrical resources to support the needed equipment?" should be addressed. Nurses can also use this form to provide a prehospital discharge visit to the home for an infant with medical technology needs. *(See Appendix J.)*
9. **Discharge Summary:** This is to be completed by the nurse at the end of care. *(See Appendix K.)*

Section 2 provides the user with forms that will be helpful in evaluating the program for effectiveness. The Case Management Log is recommended for use with infants admitted to home care after the first universal home visit. *(See Appendix L.)* Completion of the log is necessary for infants admitted to the high-risk infant follow-up program, which recommends that regularly scheduled home visits be made throught the first year for infants with significant social and or medical problems. Appendices M–Q contain forms that will be helpful in maintaining and evaluating qualitative and quantitative data.

The Bibliography preceding the Appendices will be useful in developing a resource library. The manual concludes with a list of Abbreviations, a helpful Glossary, and a detailed Index.

Department of Health and Human Services
Health Care Financing Administration

Form Approved
OMB No. 0938-0357

HOME HEALTH CERTIFICATION AND PLAN OF TREATMENT

1. Patient's HI Claim No.	2. SOC Date	3. Certification Period From: To:	4. Medical Record No.	5. Provider No.

6. Patient's Name and Address

7. Provider's Name and Address

8. Date of Birth:	9. Sex ☐ M ☐ F	10. Medications: Dose/Frequency/Route (N)ew (C)hanged

11. ICD-9-CM	Principal Diagnosis	Date

12. ICD-9-CM	Surgical Procedure	Date

13. ICD-9-CM	Other Pertinent Diagnoses	Date

14. DME and Supplies

15. Safety Measures:

16. Nutritional Req.

17. Allergies:

18.A. Functional Limitations

- 1 ☐ Amputation
- 2 ☐ Bowel/Bladder (Incontinence)
- 3 ☐ Contracture
- 4 ☐ Hearing
- 5 ☐ Paralysis
- 6 ☐ Endurance
- 7 ☐ Ambulation
- 8 ☐ Speech
- 9 ☐ Legally Blind
- A ☐ Dyspnea with Minimal Exertion
- B ☐ Other (Specify)

18.B. Activities Permitted

- 1 ☐ Complete Bedrest
- 2 ☐ Bedrest BRP
- 3 ☐ Up as Tolerated
- 4 ☐ Transfer Bed/Chair
- 5 ☐ Exercises Prescribed
- 6 ☐ Partial Weight Bearing
- 7 ☐ Independent at Home
- 8 ☐ Crutches
- 9 ☐ Cane
- A ☐ Wheelchair
- B ☐ Walker
- C ☐ No Restrictions
- D ☐ Other (Specify)

19. Mental Status

- 1 ☐ Oriented
- 2 ☐ Comatose
- 3 ☐ Forgetful
- 4 ☐ Depressed
- 5 ☐ Disoriented
- 6 ☐ Lethargic
- 7 ☐ Agitated
- 8 ☐ Other

20. Prognosis

- 1 ☐ Poor
- 2 ☐ Guarded
- 3 ☐ Fair
- 4 ☐ Good
- 5 ☐ Excellent

21. Orders for Discipline and Treatments (Specify Amount/Frequency/Duration)

22. Goals/Rehabilitation Potential/Discharge Plans

23. Verbal Start of Care and Nurse's Signature and Date Where Applicable:

24. Physician's Name and Address	25. Date HHA received Signed POT	26. I ☐ certify ☐ recertify that the above home health services are required and are authorized by me with a written plan for treatment which will be periodically reviewed by me. This patient is under my care, is confined to his home, and is in need of intermittent skilled nursing care and/or physical or speech therapy or has been furnished home health services based on such a need and no longer has a need for such care or therapy, but continues to need occupational therapy.
27. Attending Physician's Signature (required on 485 Kept on File in Medical Records of HHA)	Date Signed	

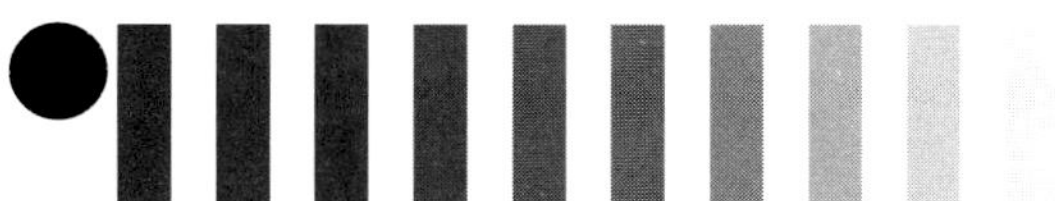

Consent for Treatment, Release of Information, Assignment of Benefits, Notice of Client Rights

Client Name: ____

Address: ____

City: ___________________________________   State: _________   Zip: _____________________

I, _________________________________ , _________________ of _________________ intending to be
    (custodial parent or legal guardian)   (relationship)   (minor client)

legally bound, hereby:

1. Consent to such care and treatment by _________________________________ , and its employees and agents (collectively, the "Agency"), as prescribed by the client's physician or dictated by the client's condition.

2. Authorize the Agency to release any medical records in its possession concerning the client as may be required by law or to pay benefits on the client's behalf. I authorize the client's physicians, insurers, and hospitals to release such medical records to the Agency at the Agency's request.

3. Authorize my insurer to disclose to the Agency the terms and extent of my coverage, and the amount of payments made to me for services provided by the Agency.

4. Assign, transfer, and set over to the Agency all of my or the client's rights to insurance proceeds or other funds to which I am or the client is or will become entitled as a result of the services rendered by the Agency.

5. Consent to and authorize payment, which would otherwise be payable to me or the client, to be made directly to the Agency. The Agency may issue a receipt for such payment which shall discharge the insurance company of its obligations under the policy to the extent of such payment.

6. Agree that I remain individually responsible to pay the Agency for all charges not paid for any reason by the insurer or other third-party payor. I understand that payment in full is due upon receipt of my bill. If payment for the Agency's services is made directly to me by my insurer, I agree to endorse the check to the provider and forward it to the Agency within three days of receipt.

A photocopy of this document, if executed, shall be considered as effective and valid as the original.

The effect of this form and the Client's Rights and Responsibilities on the back of this form have been explained to me by the Agency and I understand its content and significance.

Date: _________________   Signature: _______________________________________

Name: _______________________________________
                        (please print)

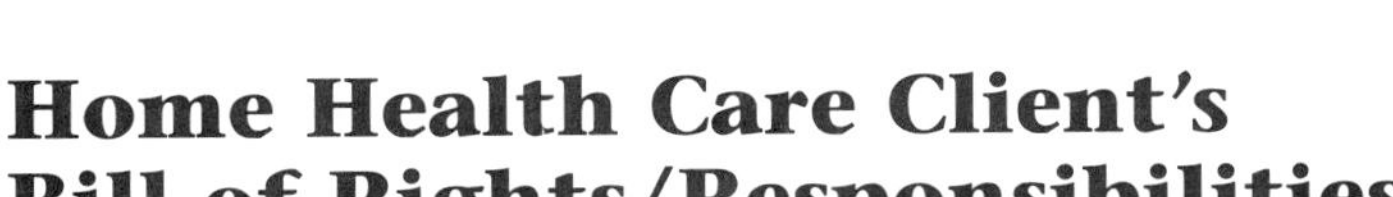

Home Health Care Client's
Bill of Rights/Responsibilities

As a home health care client you have the right to:

1. Standard: Right to be informed and to participate in planning care and treatment (1) The client has the right to be informed in advance about the care to be furnished.

2. Be given information about your rights and responsibilities for receiving home health care services, in terms and language you can reasonably expect to understand.

3. Receive a timely response from the Home Health Care Agency regarding your request for home health care services.

4. Be given information of the Home Health Care Agency charges and policy concerning payment for services, including your eligibility for third party reimbursement.

5. Choose your home health care providers.

6. Be given appropriate and professional quality home health care services without discrimination against your race, creed, color, religion, sex, national origin, sexual preference, handicap, or age.

7. The client's family or guardian may exercise the client's rights when the client has been judged incompetent.

8. The HHA must investigate complaints made by a client or the client's family or guardian regarding treatment or care that is (or fails to be) furnished, or regarding the lack of respect for the client's property by anyone furnishing services on behalf of the HHA, and must document both the existence of the complaint and the resolution of the complaint.

9. Be treated with courtesy and respect by all who provide home health care services to you; to have your property treated with respect.

10. Before the care is initiated, the HHA must inform the client, orally and in writing, of
    a. The extent of which payment may be expected from Medicare, Medicaid, or any other federally funded or aided program known to the HHA
    b. The charges for services that will not be covered by Medicare; and
    c. The charges that the individual may have to pay
    d. The client has the right to be advised orally and in writing of any changes in payment from last financial counseling.

11. The client has the right to be advised orally and in writing of any changes in payment. The HHA must advise the client of these changes orally and in writing as soon as possible, but no later than 15 working days from the date that the HHA becomes aware of a change.

12. Be given the necessary information so you will be able to give informed consent for your treatment prior to the start of any treatment.

13. Participate in the development of your home health care plan, to be informed in advance about the care to be provided and any changes in the care to be provided, including anticipated transfer of your care to another health care facility and/or termination of home health care service.

14. To be advised in advance of the disciplines that will provide care, and the frequency of visits proposed to be provided.

15. Be given data privacy and confidentiality; review your clinical record at your request.

16. Voice grievances regarding treatment or care that is (or fails to be) furnished, or regarding any lack of respect for privacy by anyone who is furnishing services on behalf of the home health care agency, without being subject to discrimination or reprisal for doing so.

   * Call _____________________ to voice a grievance and/or recommend changes in policies or services.
   * Medicare/Medicaid clients may also call a Hotline # (1-800-222-0989) to report grievances from 8:30 am–5:00 pm with answering service for non-business hours. This is *not* the number to reach the Home Health Care Agency or to obtain Medicare coverage/billing information.

17. Refuse all or part of your care to the extent permitted by law; to be informed of the expected consequences of such action.

18. The client's family or guardian may exercise the client's rights when the client has been judged incompetent.

Client Responsibilities

As a home health care client you have the responsibility to:

1. Give accurate and complete health information concerning your past illnesses, hospitalizations, medications, allergies, and other pertinent items.

2. Assist in developing and maintaining a safe environment.

3. Inform the Home Health Care Agency when you will not be able to keep a home health care visit.

4. Participate in the development and update of your home health care plan.

5. Adhere to your developed/updated home health care plan.

6. Request further information concerning anything you do not understand.

7. Give information regarding concerns and problems you have to Home Health Care Agency staff member.

Advance Directives

An advance directive is a written instruction, such as a living will or durable power of attorney for health care, recognized under state law, relating to the provision of health care when an individual's condition makes him/her unable to express his/her wishes. The intent of these provisions is to enhance an individual's control over medical treatment decisions.

The Agency's policy regarding implementation of a client's advance directive is to comply to the best of its ability with those instructions.

1. The client has been informed of the state living will law.   Yes _____   No _____

2. Does the client have a living will?   Yes _____   No _____

3. If so, is there a copy of the advance directive in the client's medical record?   Yes _____   No _____

Client Signature: __________________________________   Date: ____________________

Newborn Universal Home Risk Assessment Form

Current Medical Profile

Client Name: _________________________________ Date of Birth: _______________

Address: _____________________________________ Phone: ( ) _______________

Primary Physician: _______________________________

Physician Address: ___________________________________ Phone: ( ) _______________

Primary Diagnosis: _____________________ Secondary Diagnosis: _______________________

Allergies: _____________________ Functional Limitations: _____________________

Client's Primary Caregiver: _______________ Relationship: _______________ Health Status: _______________

Language: _______________ Race: _______________ Emergency Contact: _______________ Phone: _______________

Insurance: _______________ ID #: _______________ Caseworker: _______________ Phone: _______________

If no Insurance, why? ____

CHILD ASSESSMENT		NORM.	ABNORM.	DESCRIBE/MEASURE/PAST MEDICAL HISTORY
SKIN	Color/Condition/Cord			
METABOLIC	TPR			
NEURO.	Sleeping/Activity reflexes/Suck			
HEENT	Fontanelles			
	Auditory/Visual Response			
CARDIOVASC.	Apical Pulse			
CHEST	Lungs			
MUSCULOSKEL.	Muscle Tone			
	Feeding Type/Amt./Freq.			
GI	Elimination			
GU	Genitalia/Anus Voiding			
NUTRITIONAL	PO/Enteral			
Status	Parenteral			
	Feeding Issues			Weight

RISK ASSESSMENT (circle risk score if applicable)

I. Life Transitions
- 2 Denial/rejection medical problem
- 1 Hx current/recent incest/rape victim
- 1 Hx infant/child chronic disability
- 1 Hx of family member death
- 1 Adoption/termination considered
- 1 Suspected domestic violence

II. Emotional Status
- 1 Hx of mental illness/mental health treat./hosp.
- 1 Unresolved grief/signif. loss
- 2 Suicidal ideation
- 1 Feels isolation/alone/inadeq. support system
- 1 Questionable coping
- 1 Hx of postpartum depression
- 1 Evidence of low self-esteem

III. Substance Abuse/Risk-Taking Behaviors
- 3 Current/recent abuse of ETOH
- 3 Current/recent abuse of street drugs
- 3 Current/recent abuse of presc. meds
- 1 Law enforcement involvement
- 1 Sexual risk-taking behaviors
- 1 Tobacco use or 2nd-hand smoke exposure

IV. Parenting issues (observed/expressed)
- 1 Teen/inexperienced parent
- 1 Develop. issues (child/fam. expectations)
- 1 Discipline issues
- 1 Relationship issues (bond/nurturing)
- 1 Hx child abuse/neglect, now resolved
- 2 Child abuse/neglect, current
- 1 3 Or more children < 6 yrs. of age

V. Educational/Cultural Factors
- 1 Low literacy/limited intellectual ability
- 1 Cognitive deficits
- 1 Language barriers
- 1 Ed. level l2th or less
- 2 Ed. level 10th or less
- 3 Ed. level 9th or less or < 17 y.o.
- 1 Culture/Beliefs

VI. Economic/Resource Needs
- 1 Insuff. income to meet basic needs
- 1 No transportation
- 2 Inadequate food
- 1 Legal needs
- 2 Chronic difficulty accessing "system"
- 1 Child care problems
- 1 Medicaid problems

VII. Medical/Nutritional Factors
2 Abnl. phys. fndgs. this assess.
3 Prenatal exp. to drugs/alcohol
2 Anemia
1 Failure to thrive in sibs., prev. or existing
2 Dx or suspected malabsorption
2 Symptoms of intolerance to formula
2 Diarrhea
2 GE reflux
3 Low birth weight infant < 1500 gm

2 Problem establishing breastfeeding
3 Inadequate prenatal. care
___ immunization over 2 mos. behing due to no pediatric provider visits

1 Previous hosp. of sibs. in 1 st yr.
3 Extended hospitalization
2 Medical problems
3 Low birth weight infant < 2500 gm
2 STD exp. in preg., untreated
1 Lead exposure

VIII. Environmental
1 Housing
1 Utilities
1 Refrigeration
1 Water/sewer
1 High risk/unsafe neighborhood
1 Inadeq. prep. for infant

2 STD exp. in preg., untreated

SAFETY ASSESSMENT | YES | NO | COMMENTS

Teaching: Basic Home Safety?

CPR Training Reviewed/Reinforced?

Reviewed plan for emergency medical situation/emergency phone numbers?

Is "do not resuscitate" order applicable?

Reviewed safety instruction related to equipment and care being provided?

Physical/psychosocial environment adequate for patient care?

Other medical personnel providing care (specify name and phone): _______________________

List equipment in home/specify instructions for use given: _______________________

Reason for visit/home care needs: _______________________

Nursing diagnosis(es): _______________________

Short-term goals(s): _______________________

Long-term goals(s): _______________________

Nursing interventions (treatment, teaching, etc.): _______________________

Evaluation (response to interventions): _______________________

Referrals: _______________________

Date and Nursing Care Plan for next visit: _______________________
Communication to physician/Agency Office/Other: _______________________
Change in orders/Change in medication: _______________________
(specify change and attach completed physician verbal order form)

RN Signature: _______________________ License #: _______________ Date: ___________

Current Medication Profile

Client Name: ____   Allergies: ______________________________________

MEDICATION (Dose, Frequency, Rate)	MODIFICATION SINCE DATE OF REFERRAL	PURPOSE	SIGNIFICANT SIDE EFFECTS	INSTRUCTION *	UNDERSTANDING **

PHARMACY: ____   PHONE: ____________________

* INSTRUCTION CODES:	
1—Verbal Instructions given	4—Side effects/adverse reactions reviewed
2—Medication Sheet left in home	5—Dose & frequency reviewed
3—Medication Sheet & verbal instructions given	6—Purpose instructed
	7—All of the above

** G—Good   F—Fair   P—Poor

Nursing Plan of Care and Progress Record

CLIENT NAME: ______________________________

ADDRESS: ______________________________

____

____

PHONE: (___) ______________________________

ALLERGIES: ______________________________

HHA Supervisory Visit   Yes _____   No _____
PT satisfied with care?   Yes _____   No _____
HHA Following Care Plan   Yes _____   No _____
Care plan updated?   Yes _____   No _____

HHA's name ______________________________

LEAD SCREENING STATUS
1. Is infant the appropriate age for lead screening? Yes _____   No _____
2. If yes, does caregiver know if it was done? Yes _____   No _____
3. Does caregiver know results? Yes _____   No _____

IMMUNIZATION STATUS
1. Did infant receive any immunizations at last visit?   Yes _____   No _____
2. Has infant received any immunizations since birth?   Yes _____   No _____
3. If yes, when and which ones? (if changed from last visit): ______________________________
   Name of last pediatric provider: ______________________________
4. Is infant appropriately immunized (as reported by caregiver)?   Yes _____   No _____
5. If no, why? (as explained by caregiver): ______________________________
Date of last appt.: _________   Date of next appt.: _________

SKILLED OBSERVATION/ASSESSMENT

	Normal	Abnormal	Describe		Normal	Abnormal	Describe
Metabolic (TPR)				Genitourinary			
HEENT				Musculoskeletal			
Cardiovascular				Neurological			
Respiratory				Integumentary			
ABD/G.I.				Psychosocial			
Nutrition/Wt.				Other			

Medical Diagnosis: ______________________________

Reason for Visit/Homecare Needs: ______________________________

Nursing Diagnosis(es): ______________________________

Short-Term Goal(s): ______________________________

Long-Term Goal(s): ______________________________

Nursing Interventions (treatment, teaching, etc.): ______________________________

____

____

Evaluation (response to interventions): ______________________________

____

____

Date and Nursing Care Plan for next visit: ______________________________

____

Communication to M.D./Agency Office/Other: ______________________________

Changes in orders/changes in medication: ______________________________
(specify change and attach completed verbal order form)

RN Signature: ______________________________   License #: ______________________________   Date: _________

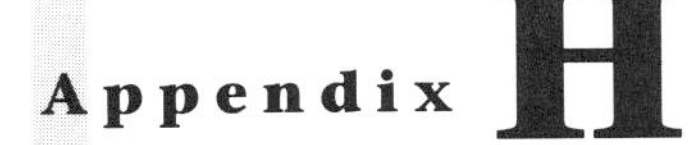

Nursing Progress Notes

Client Name: ____

DATE	

Pediatric Intake and Output Record for Parents' Use

Client Name: _______________________________________

	Date/Day	Feeding Amt & Time	Amt & Time	Amt & Time	Amt & Time	Amt & Time	Amt & Time	Amt & Time	Total # of Feedings/ per day	Wet Diapers (Mark with X for each change)	Total # of wet diapers/day (void/cc)	BM
MONDAY												
TUESDAY												
WEDNESDAY												
THURSDAY												
FRIDAY												
SATURDAY												
SUNDAY												
MONDAY												
TUESDAY												
WEDNESDAY												
THURSDAY												
FRIDAY												
SATURDAY												
SUNDAY												

Home Care Needs Assessment Tool

CLIENT

Name: _________________________________ Client's DOB: _______________ Client's Age: _________

Client's Ins. #: _________________________________ Clients SS#: _________________________________

Client's Race: _________________ Client's Sex: _________

Current Telephone #: (   ) _________________________ Current Telephone #: (   ) _________________________

INSTITUTION: _________________________________

_______ Home   _______ Shelter   _______ Homeless   _______ Staying with Relatives

Address: ____
(street)   (apt.)   (City)   (Zip)

EMERGENCY CONTACT PERSONS

Name: _________________________________ Relationship: _________________ Age: _________

Phone: _________________

Address: ____
(street)   (apt.)   (City)   (Zip)

MOTHER'S DATA

Name: _________________________________ Phone: _________________ Age: _________________

Address: ____
(street)   (apt.)   (City)   (Zip)

Best Time to Contact: _________________________________

FATHER'S DATA

Name: _________________________________ Phone: _________________ Age: _________________

Address: ____
(street)   (apt.)   (City)   (Zip)

Best Time to Contact: _________________________________

CHILD'S DOCTOR (must use PCP if applicable)

Name: _______________________________   Hospital: _______________________   Phone: _______________

Address: ____
              (street)   (apt.)   (City)   (Zip)

CONSULTING DOCTORS ON CARE

1. _______________________________   _______________________________
              (Name)   (Phone)

2. _______________________________   _______________________________
              (Name)   (Phone)

3. _______________________________   _______________________________
              (Name)   (Phone)

OTHER CONSULTANTS

SW: _______________________________   _______________________________
             (Name)   (Phone)

Other: _______________________________   _______________________________
             (Name)   (Phone)

DIAGNOSES

1. _______________________________   2. _______________________________

3. _______________________________

Exacerbating potentials: ____

I. BIRTH DATA

1. Hospital of Delivery: _______________________________

2. History of Prenatal Care: _______________________________

3. Gestational Age at Birth: _______________   Wgt.: _______________

     Problems: ____

4. Delivery: _______ Vaginal   _______ C-Section

5. Condition of Baby at Delivery/Complications

II. CURRENT STATE OF HEALTH

1. Physical

2. Mental

3. Emotional

4. Social

5. Hospitalizations/Surgeries

III. CHILD'S HEALTH CARE NEEDS: (Specify with as much detail as possible)

1. Diet/Feeding Schedule:

2. Activity:

3. Physical Therapy:

4. Psychological Therapy/OT:

5. Educational Therapies:

6. Speech Therapy:

7. Equipment and use including tubes present—source of equipment—who supplies:

8. Medications—name, dose, route, freq., purpose:

9. Teaching Needed:

_____ Nutrition	_____ Community resources	_____ Respite
_____ Growth/dev.	_____ Utilities	_____ Others
_____ Formula prep and access to formula	_____ Phone	
_____ Parenting education	_____ Housing	
_____ Budgeting of financial resources	_____ Cooking	
_____ Home safety	_____ Water	
_____ Parenting		

10. Referrals already made: ____

11. Referrals needed: ____

      _____ Kencrest   _____ Other

IV. FAMILY DATA/SUPPORT NETWORK

1. Primary Caretaker of Child

    Name: ___________________________________

    Health Status: ___________________________________

    Ed. Issues: ___________________________________

    Age: _________

2. Siblings (Name, Age, Address, Medical Issues, Parents):

_______ no. of Siblings:

3. Other Household Members (Name, Age, Medical Issues):

4. Other Significant Others/Extended Family Members. Are they available to assist with care of child—when?

5. Summary of Household Function—Do people work together? Do they get along, who is in charge, etc.:

6. Evidence of Drug/alcohol Use:

V. HOUSING INFORMATION:

1. Current Residence: _____ permanent _____ temporary

2. Type of Residence: _____ sngle Family _____ apt. _____ shelter

3. Length of Time in Current Residence: __________

4. Are there Plans for Move? _____ Yes _____ When? _____ No

   New Address: __________________________________

5. Layout of House: _______ no. of Bedrooms _______ no. of Bathrooms _______ kitchen
   _______ living Area _______ furniture _______ dining Area

   Condition of House: ____

6. Safety issues at House:

   Outlets: _____ 2-prong _____ 3-prong _____ adeq. No.'s _____ inadeq. No.'s

   Smoke Alarms: Yes _____ No _____ no. of alarms: _____

   Stable Railings: Yes _____ No _____

   Adequate Lighting: Yes _____ No _____ Specify: _____________________________

   Emergency No.'s Posted: Yes _____ No _____

   Sanitation: No. of Bathrooms: _______

   A. Is kitchen sanitary: Yes _____ No _____ Specify: ____________________________

   B. Pest Control: Are the following present:

   _____ roaches _____ rats/Mice _____ flies

   C. Plumbing problems __________________________________

Medication storage—specify plan for storage, if refrigeration needed:

Infection control needs surrounding care:

7. Will house need modification/rearrangement for child (specify):

8. Specify space child will have to sleep, play, exercise, etc., and equipment (bed, toys) available:

VI.   FINANCIAL DATA

1. Source of income for parent/guardian   Name: _______________________________________

_______ DPA   Amount $ ___________________   _______ SSI   Amount $ ___________________

_______ Job   Amount $ ___________________

_______ Other: Specify type/amount: ____

_______ Child Support   Amount $ ___________________

2. Income Supplements—Program Participation

_______ WIC   _______ Food Stamps $ ___________________

_______ Public housing   Rent $ ___________________

_______ Section VIII housing   Amount $ ___________________

_______ School lunch   _______ School breakfast

3. Expenses—Specify Amount

_______ Rent $ ___________________   _______ Food $ ___________________

_______ Utilities $ ___________________   _______ Meds $ ___________________

_______ Trans. $ ___________________   _______ Clothing $ ___________________

4. HEALTH INSURANCE:

_______ MA   _______ HMA   _______ NONE   _______ Other: ___________________

_______ NEEDS ASSIST—Specify:

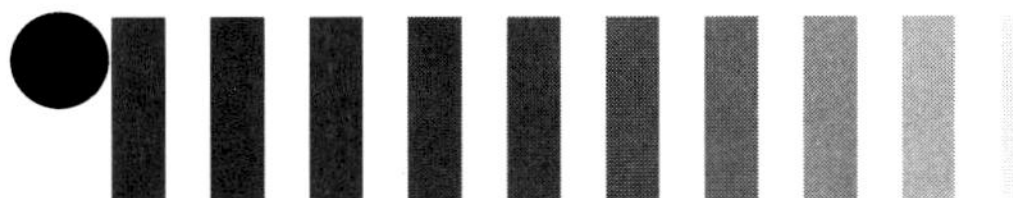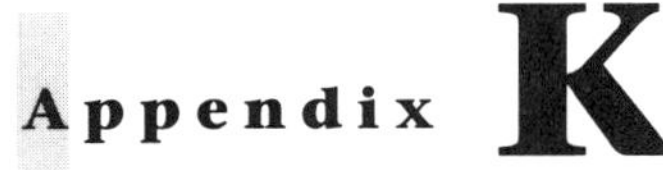

Discharge Summary

Client Name: _______________________________ Date of Birth: _______________________________

Insurance Co.: _______________________________ ID#: _______________________________

Address: ____

Diagnosis: ____

Date of First Visit: _____________________ Date of Last Visit: _____________________

No. of Visits: RN: ______ LPN: ______ PT: ______ OT: ______ ST: ______ HHA: ______ Other: _______________
(type of service)

Date of Discharge: _____________________

Initiation of Discharge: Physician (give name): ____

Physician's Address: ____

Agency: _____________________ Client/Family: _____________________

Reason for termination of service: ____

____

Summary of Progress and Client/Patient Status at Discharge (Physical, Mental, Emotional):

SUBJECTIVE: ____

____

____

OBJECTIVE: ____

____

ASSESSMENT: ____

____

____

                                                          ATTAINED

GOALS: _______________________________ Yes: ________ No: ________

_______________________________ Yes: ________ No: ________

_______________________________ Yes: ________ No: ________

PLAN
Referrals made and final disposition: ____

____

____

Client/Patient notified of discharge: Yes: ______ No: ______ Family notified of discharge: Yes: ______ No: ______

Physician notified of discharge: Yes: ______ No: ______

Signature: _______________________________ Date: _____________________

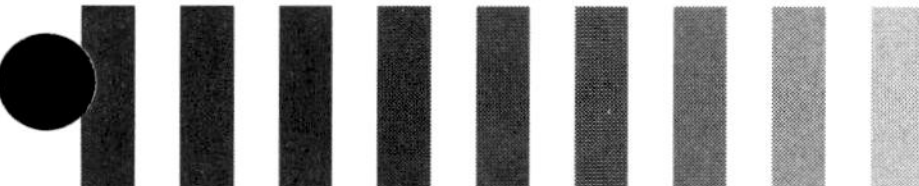

High-Risk Follow-Up Program Case Management Log

Measureable Outcomes—Plan of Care Goals

Process (date/time of appointments):

Completed:

PLAN	OUTCOME	COMMENTS

BIRTH–2 MONTHS

At least 1 Newborn Visit to
 pediatric provider

HBV given

Health insurance for
 newborn

Appt. w/caseworker to enroll baby
 by 2nd wk of age

    Emergency

    Urgent care

    Routine

Social and financial support

Food resources

Adequate maternal foods/fluid

Adequate newborn resources

Food stamps

WIC referral

Mental health, drug/alcohol
 counseling

Newborn wt. gain of 4–6 oz/wk

Linkage to health care system initiated

Transp. avail. for medical care appts.

Insurance provider to initiate
 newborn enrollment

WIC appts.

PLAN	OUTCOME	COMMENTS

ER use and rehosp. prevented

Parenting problems identified and
  referral or teaching initiated

2–4 MONTHS

Newborn adequately nourished
  as evidenced by growth and
  wt. gain

> Developmental milestones
>   reached by age 3 months
>
> Raise head and chest when
>   lying on stomach
>
> Stretch legs and kick when
>   lying down
>
> Bring hands and toys to
>   mouth
>
> Reach for dangling objects
>
> Grasp and shake toys like
>   rattles
>
> Recognize familiar objects and
>   people
>
> Follow moving objects with eyes
>
> Watch your facial expression
>
> Smile and babble
>
> Enjoy people, including
>   strangers
>
> Linkages to health care
>
> Brute. in place
>
> Pediatric provider appt. for
>   immunizations kept

At 2 months DPT–polio, HIB

At 4 mos. DPT–polio, HIB

Lead level determined

Referrals previously initiated in place

EPSDT program

4–6 MONTHS

Growth adequate for age

> Developmental milestones reached
>   by age 6 mos.
>
> Work hard to get objects that are
>   out of reach
>
> Find partially hidden toys
>
> Respond to own name and
>   familiar words
>
> Babble in response to your speech

PLAN	OUTCOME	COMMENTS

Sit with help

Roll stomach to back

Reach for and grab toys

Pediatric provider appt. for
  immunizations kept

At 6 months. DPT–polio, HIB, HBV

Lead level drawn at 6 mos and
  result known

Nutritional support and
  teaching

Adequate food available

Transition from all formula to
  baby foods started

Follow-up with community
  resource linkages to which
  family previously referred

6–8 MONTHS

Growth adequate for age

Developmental milestones
  reached

Any outstanding problems
  previously listed

8–10 MONTHS

Lead level drawn by 9 mos.
  if first result was >10–14 µg/dl

Any outstanding problems
  previously listed

10–12 MONTHS

Lead level drawn by 12 mos.
  if first result was < 10 µg/dl

Any outstanding problems
  previously listed

Discharge Planning

Record Audit Form for Collection of High-Risk Newborn Follow-Up Data

Newborn Name: _______________________________   Date of Service: _________________

ADM: _________________   D/C: _________________   No. of visits: _________________

Describe problems in carrying out plan of care: _______________________________________

____

____

Is it known if client has working phone? Yes _______   No _______

Was newborn difficult to locate at times? If yes, describe: _____________________________

____

____

Do there appear to be language barriers: Yes _______   No _______

Do notes reflect dates of newborn's pediatric appointments? Yes _______   No _______

Describe: ____

____

Do notes reflect if newborn attended pediatric appointments? Yes _______   No _______

Do notes reflect illnesses which may have delayed immunizations or gotten infant off traditional schedule?

    Yes _______   No _______

Is there a data outcome form retrievable for this newborn? Yes _______   No _______

Describe any insurance changes: ____

Do notes reflect primary care at any other location? Yes _______   No _______

Immunization status:

	Up to date	Not up to date
DPT:	_______	_______
OPY:	_______	_______
HIB:	_______	_______
HBV:	_______	_______
TB:	_______	_______

High-Risk Newborn Follow-Up Program

Chart Review

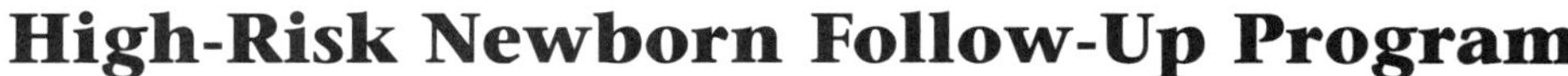

Name: _______________________________   Date: _________________

Admission date: ________________   Insurance type at admission: ________________

Discharge date: ________________   Insurance type at discharge: ________________

Length of service (wks): ________________   Total no. of visits: ________________

Hospital admission: Yes _______   No _______

Dates and Diagnosis: ____

ER Visit: Yes _______   No _______

Dates and Diagnosis: ____

REASON FOR DISCHARGE:

Not home for Scheduled Visit __________   Newborn Death (home) __________

Refused visit(s) __________   Insurer denied authorization __________

Moved/unable to locate __________   Improved condition/stable __________

Newborn Hospitalized __________   Noncompliant __________

Other: ____

Newborn Quantitative Data

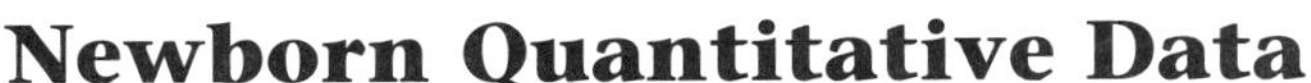

Monthly and quarterly data collection: Disposition of newborn referrals

Universal newborn screenings

Newborn referrals: _________

    No. refused visit: _________

    No. unable to locate: _________

    No. ineligible per ins. co.: _________

    No. misc. (no-show, moved, hosp, foster placement): _________

Total no. not visited of referrals made: _________

Total no. newborns seen: _________

Total no. cases visited and opened for follow-up of risk factors identified at hospital discharge or newborn home visit other than high-risk admission criteria: _________

    No. newborns: _________

    No. visits: _________

Total no. cases opened for follow-up of high-risk admission criteria

    No. newborns: _________

    No. visits: _________

    No. newborns remaining in service after 62 days:

    No prenatal care: _________

    Teen < 17 years old: _________

    Substance abuse: _________

    Lack of adequate prenatal care: _________

    Other: _________

Newborn Qualitative Data

Total # newborns seen ________

________ Reports of illness or changes in condition by nurse to practitioner

________ Emergency room visits

________ Rehospitalizations

________ Identification of primary care for follow-up

________ Identification of WIC

________ Identification of insurance

________ No. newborns meeting high risk admission criteria

________ No. newborns followed in home care beyond 62 days meeting high risk admission criteria

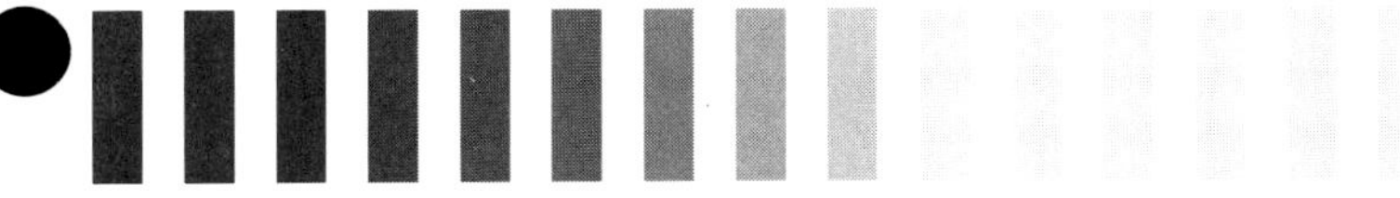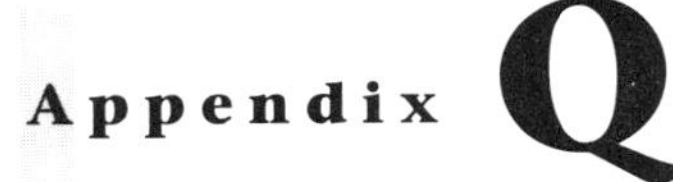

Outcome Data for Newborns in High-Risk Follow-Up

Patient Name: _________________________________   DOS: _________________

Admission Date: _________________   Pediatric F/U Site: _________________________________

Birth Weight: _________

Appropriate for Age

Weights: 3 mos   _______ Y _______ N _______ NA

                6 mos   _______ Y _______ N _______ NA

                9 mos   _______ Y _______ N _______ NA

            12 mos   _______ Y _______ N _______ NA

Lead Screen done at or by age 6 mos.: _______ Y _______ N _______ NA

Lead Level: _____________   Plan for followup (if applicable):

Other important data regarding illness (explain):

Illness: _______ Y _______ N

ER Visit: _______ Y _______ N

Hospitalization: _______ Y _______ N

Referrals to Child Protective Service: _______ Y _______ N

Transfer to another pediatric provider for follow-up:

_______ Y (specify name): _________________________________   N _______

Unable to determine follow-up site: _______ Y _______ N

IMMUNIZATIONS (LIST ALL DATES):

DPT: _______ Y _______ N _______ NA

Oral Polio Vaccine: _______ Y _______ N _______ NA

MMR: _______ Y _______ N _______ NA

HIS: _______ Y _______ N _______ NA

HIBV: _______ Y _______ N _______ NA

TB: _______ Y _______ N _______ NA

Other: _______ Y _______ N _______ NA

Appropriately immunized for age: _______ Y _______ N

Common Abbreviations in Maternal–Child Nursing

ABC	alternative birthing center; airway, breathing, circulation
AC	abdominal circumference
ADA	American Diabetes Association
ADL	activities of daily living
AFP	alpha-fetoprotein
AFV	amniotic fluid volume
AGA	average for gestational age
AIDS	acquired immune deficiency syndrome
AROM	artificial rupture of membranes
BAT	brown adipose tissue (brown fat)
BGS	blood glucose sample
bili	blood bilirubin level
BL	baseline (fetal heart rate baseline)
BMR	basal metabolic rate
BOW	bag of waters
BP	blood pressure
BPD	biparietal diameter; bronchopulmonary dysplasia
BPM	beats per minute
BSE	breast self-examination
BUN	blood urea nitrogen
CC	chest circumference; cord compression; chief complaint
cc	cubic centimeter
CDC	Centers for Disease Control
CF	cystic fibrosis
CHF	congestive heart failure
CID	cytomegalic inclusion disease
CMV	cytomegalovirus
cm	centimeter
CNM	certified nurse-midwife
CNS	central nervous system
CPAP	continuous positive airway pressure
CPD	cephalopelvic disproportion; citrate–phosphate–dextrose
CPR	cardiopulmonary resuscitation
C/S	cesarean section or c-section
DD	developmental disability
DHS	Department of Health Services
dil	dilatation
D&C	dilatation and curettage
DES	diethylstilbestrol
DFMR	daily fetal movement response

DM	diabetes mellitus
DNR	do not resucitate
DOB	date of birth
DRG	diagnostic related groups
DTR	deep tendon reflexes
ECMO	extracorporeal membrane oxygenator
EDC	estimated date or confinement
EFA	essential fatty acid
EFM	electronic fetal monitoring
EFW	estimated fetal weight
EI	early intervention
EPIS	episiotomy
FAD	fetal activity diary
FAS	fetal alcohol syndrome
FBS	fetal blood sample; fasting blood sugar
FBM	fetal breathing movements
FHR	fetal heart rate
FHT	fetal heart tones
FM	fetal movement
FMD	fetal movement diary
FMR	fetal movement record
FPG	fasting plasma glucose
FTT	failure to thrive
G&D	growth and development
GDM	gestational diabetes mellitus
GI	gastrointestinal
GRAV	gravida
GT	gastrostomy tube
GTT	glucose tolerance test
GYN	gynecology
HAL	hyperalimentation
HCG	human chorionic gonadotrophin
HEENT	head, ears, eyes, nose, throat
HIV	human immunodeficiency virus
IDDM	insulin-dependent diabetes mellitus
IGT	impaired glucose tolerance
IL	intralipids
ITP	idiopathis thrombocytopenic purpura
IUFD	intrauterine fetal demise
IUGR	intrauterine growth retardation
IV	intravenous
JCAHO	Joint Commission for the Accreditation of Healthcare Organizations
L/S ratio	lecithin/sphingomyelin ratio
MAP	mean arterial pressure
MCH	maternal–child health
MH	mental health
MR	mental retardation
NG	nasogastric tube
NIDDM	non–insulin-dependent diabetes mellitus
NKA	no know allergies
NPO	nulla per os
NSCT	nipple stimulation challenge test
NST	non-stress test
OB	obstetric
OCT	oxytocin challenge test

OES	oral electrolyte solution
ORS	oral rehydration solution
ORT	oral rehydration therapy
Peds	pediatrids
PIH	pregancy-induced hypertension
PO	per os (by mouth)
PROM	premature rupture of membranes
RBC	red blood cell
RDS	Respiratory distress syndrome
RMA	right mentoanterior
ROA	right occiput anterior
ROM	rupture of membranes
ROP	right occiput posterior
ROP	retinopathy of prematurity
ROT	right occiput transverse
RMP	right mentoposterior
RMT	right mentotransverse
RSA	right sacroanterior
RSP	right sacroposterior
SFD	small for dates
SGA	small for gestational age
SIDS	sudden infant death syndrome
SOAP	subjective data, objective data, analysis, plan
SOB	short of breath
SROM	spontaneous rupture of the membranes
S/S	signs and symptoms
STD	sexually transmitted disease
TORCH	toxoplasmosis, other (viruses) rubella, cytomegalovirus, herpes virus type 2
TPN	total parenteral nutrition
TSS	toxic shock syndrome
U/A	urinalysis
UAC	umbilical artery catheter
UC	uterine contraction
UPI	uteroplacental insufficiency
UTI	urinary tract infection
VBAC	vaginal birth after cesarean
WBC	white blood cell
WIC	supplemental food program for woman, infants, and children
WNL	within normal limits

Glossary

abortion	loss of pregnancy before the fetus is viable outside the uterus; miscarriage, or elective termination
abruptio placentae	partial or total premature separation of a normally implanted placenta.
acrocyanosis	cyanosis of the extremities
albinism	a congenital absence of normal skin pigmentation
albuminuria	readily detectable amounts of albumin in the urine
amniocentesis	removal of amniotic fluid by insertion of needle into the amniotic sac (amniotic fluid is used to assess health and maturity status of fetus)
amnion	the inner of the two uterine membranes that form the sac containing the fetus and the amniotic fluid
amniotic fluid	the fluid surrounding the fetus in utero
amnionitis	infection within the amniotic fluid
amniotomy	the artificial rupturing of the amniotic sac
analgesic	drug that relieves pain
anencephaly	congenital deformity in which the cerebrum, cerebellum, and flat bones of the skull are absent
anesthesia	partial or complete loss of sensation with or without loss of consciousness; excess amount of carbon dioxide in the body
anomaly	a malformation; an organ or structure
anoxia	deficiency of oxygen
antepartum	time between conception and the onset of labor
anterior	pertaining to the front
Apgar score	a scoring system used to evaluate newborns at 1 minute and 5 minutes after delivery. The total score is derived by assessing five signs: heart rate, respiratory effort, muscle tone, reflex irritability, and color
apnea	a condition that occurs when respirations cease for more than 20 seconds, with cyanosis
Bartholin's glands	two small mucus glands on each side of the vaginal orifice that secrete small amounts of mucus during intercourse
bilirubin	orange or yellowish pigment in bile; a breakdown product of red blood cells that is carried by the blood to the liver, where it is excreted in the bile and in the stools.
brown adipose tissue	fat deposits in neonates that provide greater heat protection

cephalhematoma	subcutaneous swelling found on the head of an infant several days after delivery
cephalic	referring to the head
chorion	one of the two uterine membranes closest to the intrauterine wall
mastitis	inflammation of the breast
neonatal mortality rate	number of deaths of infants in the first 28 days of life per 1,000 live births
neonate	infant from birth through the first 28 days of life
neonatology	the specialty that focuses on the management of high-risk conditions of the newborn
omphalitis	infection of the umbilicus
omphalocele	congential herniation of abdominal contents into the base of the umbilicus
outlet dystocia	inadequate pelvic size, causing the fetal head to be pushed backward toward the coccyx, making delivery of head difficult
ovum	female reproductive cell; egg
oxygen toxicity	serious, sometimes irreversible damage to pulmonary capillary endothelium associated with excessive levels of oxygen therapy
palpation	use of fingers or hands to manually perform assessment
perforation of the uterus	a hole made in the uterus
periodic breathing	sporadic episodes of apnea, not associated with cyanosis, lasting about 10 seconds
persistent pulmonary hypertension	a neonatal syndrome secondary to pulmonary hypertension; seen in preterm but more frequently in full-term and postmature infants
phenylketonuria (PKU)	a recessive hereditary metabolic error that causes the buildup of phenylalanine, leading to mental retardation, brain damage, light pigmentation and other growth deformities. It is treated with a low-phenylalanine diet
phlebitis	inflammation of a vein
phototherapy	treatment of newborn jaundice by exposure to natural or special artificial light
physiologic jaundice	harmless condition caused by the normal reduction of red blood cells, occurs usually between the second and fifth day after birth, peaking on the fifth to seventh day, and disappearing between the seventh and tenth day.
preterm infant	any infant born before 37 weeks' gestation
preterm labor	labor beginning before the 37th week of gestation
postmature infant	a newborn that is overly developed or that is more than 42 weeks' gestation
postnatal	occurring after birth
precipitous delivery	unduly rapid progression of labor
preeclampsia	toxemia of pregnancy; characterized by hypertension, albuminuria, and edema
pregnancy-induced hypertension (PIH)	a hypertensive disorder including preeclampsia and identified by the three cardinal signs: hypertension, edema, and proteinuria

prolapsed cord umbilical cord that becomes compressed in the vagina before the fetus is delivered, resulting in emergency situation for the fetus

prolonged labor labor lasting more than 24 hours

puerperium the period after completion of the third stage of labor until involution of the uterus is complete at about 6 weeks

rales an abnormal respiratory sound caused by air passing through fluid in the alveoli and bronchioles

regional anesthesia injection of local anesthetic

rhonchi coarse, abnormal auscultatory sounds

spina bifida occulta a defect in the vertebrae of the spinal column without protrusion of neural components

surfactant a surface-active mixture of secreted lipoproteins caused by *Candida albicans*, in the alveoli and air passages; it reduces surface tension of pulmonary fluids and contributes to the elasticity of lung tissue

tachycardia abnormally rapid heart rate

tachypnea excessively rapid respirations

term infant a liveborn infant at 38 to 42 weeks' gestation

thromboembolus thrombotic material or clot within the vein

umbilical cord the structure connecting the placenta to the umbilicus of the fetus through which the fetus receives nutrition and eliminates wastes

urinary meatus external opening of the urethra

uterus the hollow muscular organ in which the fertilized egg is implanted and in which the developing fetus is nourished until birth

vagina the musculomembranous tube located between the external genitals and the uterus

varicose veins permanently distended veins

vasectomy surgical removal of a portion of the vas deferens

Index

Note: Page numbers followed by *t* indicate tables.